Optimizing Aesthetic Toxin Results

Series in Cosmetic and Laser Therapy

About the Series

The world of cosmetic and aesthetic medicine and surgery has grown greatly in size and complexity over recent years, and the series in *Cosmetic and Laser Therapy* keeps readers up to date with the latest clinical therapies to improve and rejuvenate the appearance of skin, hair, and nails. Published in association with the *Journal of Cosmetic and Laser Therapy*, each volume in the series is preparedseparately and typically focuses on a topical theme. Volumes are published on an occasional basis,according to the emergence of new developments.

Illustrated Manual of Injectable Fillers: A Technical Guide to the Volumetric Approach to Whole Body Rejuvenation, First Edition
Neil S. Sadick, Paul J. Carniol, Deborshi Roy, Luitgard Wiest

Comprehensive Aesthetic Rejuvenation: A Regional Approach
Jenny Kim, Gary Lask, Andrew Nelson

Textbook of Chemical Peels: Superficial, Medium, and Deep Peels in Cosmetic Practice, Second Edition
Philippe Deprez, Philippe Deprez

Textbook of Cosmetic Dermatology, Fifth Edition
Robert Baran, Howard I. Maibach

Disorders of Fat and Cellulite: Advances in Diagnosis and Treatment
David J. Goldberg, Alexander L. Berlin

Botulinum Toxins in Clinical Aesthetic Practice 3E, Volume Two: Functional Anatomy and Injection Techniques
Anthony V. Benedetto

Botulinum Toxins in Clinical Aesthetic Practice 3E, Volume One: Clinical Adaptations
Anthony V. Benedetto

Botulinum Toxins in Clinical Aesthetic Practice 3E: Two Volume Set
Anthony V. Benedetto

Aesthetic Rejuvenation Challenges and Solutions: A World Perspective
Paul J. Carniol, Gary D. Monheit

Illustrated Manual of Injectable Fillers, Second Edition
Neil S. Sadick

Optimizing Aesthetic Toxin Results
Yates Yen-Yu Chao

Adapting Dermal Fillers in Clinical Practice
Yates Yen-Yu Chao, Sebastian Cotofana

For more information about this series please visit: https://www.crcpress.com/Series-in-Cosmetic-and-Laser-Therapy/book-series/CRCCOSLASTHE

Optimizing Aesthetic Toxin Results

Edited by
Yates Yen-Yu Chao

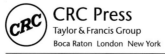

CRC Press
Taylor & Francis Group
Boca Raton London New York

CRC Press is an imprint of the
Taylor & Francis Group, an **informa** business

First edition published 2022
by CRC Press
6000 Broken Sound Parkway NW, Suite 300, Boca Raton, FL 33487-2742

and by CRC Press
2 Park Square, Milton Park, Abingdon, Oxon, OX14 4RN

Library of Congress Cataloging-in-Publication Data

Names: Chao, Yates Yen-Yu, editor.
Title: Optimizing aesthetic toxin results / edited by Yates Yen-Yu Chao.
Description: First edition. | Boca Raton, FL : CRC Press, 2021. | Includes bibliographical references and index.
Identifiers: LCCN 2021040029 (print) | LCCN 2021040030 (ebook) | ISBN 9780367441852 (hardback) | ISBN 9781032197753 (paperback) | ISBN 9781003008132 (ebook)
Subjects: MESH: Botulinum Toxins, Type A--therapeutic use | Esthetics | Off-Label Use
Classification: LCC RL120.B66 (print) | LCC RL120.B66 (ebook) | NLM QV 140 | DDC 615.7/78--dc23
LC record available at https://lccn.loc.gov/2021040029
LC ebook record available at https://lccn.loc.gov/2021040030

ISBN: 978-0-367-44185-2 (hbk)
ISBN: 978-1-032-19775-3 (pbk)
ISBN: 978-1-003-00813-2 (ebk)

DOI: 10.1201/9781003008132

Typeset in Times
by Deanta Global Publishing Services, Chennai, India

Contents

Preface

In the issue of *Time Magazine* on Botox's 30th birthday, this tiny chain of amino acid was praised as a drug that treats almost everything. The evolution of this pharmaceutical protein, like other epic stories in medical history, begins with disease and mortality and moves to sophisticated beauty. As more has been disclosed and understood about it, we can now use and administer it with precision to treat a variety of problems or to deal with something that can't be called a problem but represents the attainment of a dream.

For an injectable drug that is known and labeled as a toxin, the practice of administration has to be more or less conservative and has to follow the experience of precedents. When looking back at the beginning of teaching on aesthetic toxin practices about the location and dosage of injection, many standard protocols that prevailed for many years already look outdated now, and many understandings that were taken for granted are actually based on limited evidentiary support.

This book does not repeat the information in the many publications on toxin injection guidance and muscular anatomy but aims to remind readers of the ultimate goal of our aesthetic treatments and the responsibility of medical practitioners. The desire for beauty or attractiveness has to be weighed against the dangers inherent in achieving functional muscle paralysis. Even after so many years of experience with toxins that can block nerve and muscle connections, we need to be sufficiently clear and sure about what is involved. Every treatment by injection delivers a biological substance that can have consequences on the opponent synergistic muscles and, moreover, the whole face. It is more than a straightforward scenario about where to inject; aesthetic practice and facial alteration in contours and in functional motions amount to more than just a measurable medicine and a certain number of units. That is even more true for toxin patients who will keep on needing injection treatments more than twice a year and will probably need more in the future.

The contents of this book concern the practical use of botulinum toxin for aesthetic purposes with a high percentage of off-label usage. The format of a problem-oriented presentation has been adopted to enable quicker and more practical reference. The book begins with the insights of Prof. Michael Martin, offering more perspectives on the use of this tiny peptide as a protein pharmaceutical. Michael also gives advice in the other chapters on toxin immunology, physiology, and concerns about dermal application and combinations. Prof. Jürgen Frevert, a scholar who has devoted his career to the toxin industry, discusses the details of product manufacturing, reconstitution, comparison, and resistance. Thirdly, Sebastian Cotofana, MD, PhD, the brilliant anatomist, elaborates with more details relating to the targets of aesthetic toxin injection.

Yates Yen-Yu Chao, MD
Chao Institute of Aesthetic Medicine
Taipei, Taiwan

Contributors

Sebastian Cotofana
Department of Clinical Anatomy
Mayo Clinic College of Medicine
    and Science
Rochester, MN

Jürgen Frevert
Botulinum Toxin Research
Merz Pharmaceuticals GmbH
Potsdam, Germany

Michael Martin
Department of Immunology
Justus Liebig University
Giessen, Germany

Nicholas Moellhoff
Division of Hand, Plastic and Aesthetic Surgery
University Hospital
LMU Munich
Munich, Germany

Introduction: Injectable Botulinum Toxin and Its Aesthetic Applications

Michael Martin

The biopharmaceutical BoNT/A1 is a protein of bacterial origin that acts selectively on synaptic nerve terminals in the periphery by inhibiting the release of the neurotransmitter acetylcholine. The favorable pharmacological properties include high selectivity, very high potency, and, most importantly, the reversibility of the "neurotoxic" effect. This makes BoNT/A1 a very versatile and clinically valuable drug for a continuously growing number of clinical indications but especially in aesthetic medicine, with more than 7.4 million applications in 2018 in the USA alone. All BoNT/A1 pharma proteins presently on the market are manufactured by fermentation of *Clostridium botulinum* and subsequent purification of the pharma protein from bacterial lysates.

In nature, BoNT/A1 is a food poison that is normally ingested when eating contaminated food. Being a protein, BoNT/A1 needs protection from digestive enzymes in the gastrointestinal tract. This explains why bacteria produce it as a large complex with a series of proteins that protect it and facilitate its uptake into the tissue.

THE NEUROTOXIN: BoNT/A1

The minimal pharmacologically active substance BoNT/A1 is a relatively large protein of 150 kDa consisting of an N-terminal light chain of 50 kDa and a C-terminal heavy chain of 100 kDa, covalently linked by a disulfide bond (Figure 0.1). The two C-terminal subdomains of the heavy chain are involved in binding to and uptake into the nerve terminal, whereas the N-terminal subdomain is responsible for the translocation of the light chain into the cytosol. The light chain is a Zn^{2+}-dependent protease that cleaves SNAP25, a molecule essential for fusing presynaptic vesicles with the plasma membrane at the nerve terminal.

THE FOOD POISON: BoNT/A1 WITHIN THE LARGE PROGENITOR TOXIN COMPLEX (L-PTC)

The non-toxin non-hemagglutinin protein (NTNHA) and three differently sized hemagglutinins are neurotoxin-associated proteins contained in the food poison (*and many – but not all – drug formulations*). NTNHA binds closely to BoNT/A and shields it from digestive enzymes in the gastrointestinal tract. In addition, it plays the role of connection to the triskelion formed by the hemagglutinins (Figure 0.2 upper panel). L-PTC is stable in the acidic environment of the stomach and gut (pH below 6) and remains intact. Coming from the gut lumen, the neurotoxin must

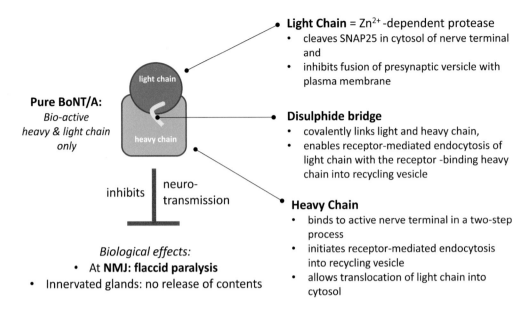

FIGURE 0.1 Scheme of minimal pharmacologically active BoNT/A neurotoxin. Pure and bio-active botulinum neurotoxin A consists of a 25 kDa light chain and a 50 kDa heavy chain covalently linked by a disulfide bridge (yellow line). This complex is sufficient to achieve the desired pharmacological effects if injected into the tissue of a patient including flaccid paralysis at the neuromuscular junction (NMJ). These effects are based on the inhibition of the release of the neurotransmitter acetylcholine from presynaptic vesicles in the periphery, resulting in the blocking of neurotransmission in the affected nerve terminal.

make its way into the lymph and blood stream in order to reach peripheral nerve cells. This uptake is facilitated by the hemagglutinins (HA), a total of three differently sized proteins that interact in a defined manner to form a complex structure that resembles a triskelion (Figure 0.2 upper panel). Pure BoNT/A1 is unable to cross epithelial or endothelial barriers (such as the blood–brain barrier).

FATE OF THE COMPLEX ENTRY INTO THE TISSUE: RELEASE OF BoNT/A1

Leaving the acidic gut lumen, BoNT/A1 faces a neutral or slightly basic pH. This results in the immediate dissociation of the pH-sensitive complex into BoNT/A1 and a neurotoxin-free complex (Figure 0.2 lower panel). This is true for the food poison *and* pharmaceuticals that contain BoNT/A1 within the L-PTC. BoNT/A1 reaches the interstitial fluid alone where it is collected by the lymphatic system. Together with the lymph, BoNT/A1 is delivered to the blood to be distributed around the body.

Pharmaceutical BoNT/A1 is injected into the tissue. Bio-active BoNT/A, consisting of heavy and light chains linked by the disulfide bond, alone suffices to achieve the desired pharmacological effects. There is neither need nor function for further bacterial proteins.

In the past several myths have "evolved" claiming that complexing proteins stabilize BoNT/A1 in formulations or influence the pharmacology of the pharma protein. More recent data convincingly show that they play no such beneficial role. In contrast, they carry the risk of increasing the immunogenicity of the drug (see Chapter 1).

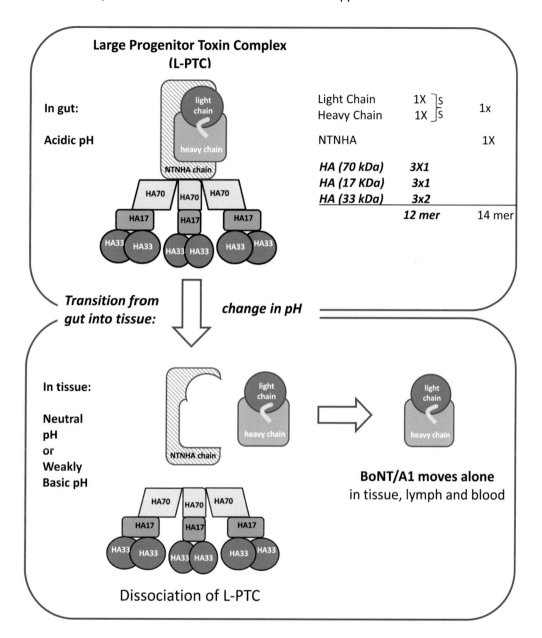

FIGURE 0.2   Scheme of large progenitor toxin complex (L-PTC). At the acidic pH in stomach and gut, botulinum neurotoxin A is part of a large progenitor toxin complex (L-PTC), consisting of a total of 14 individual proteins (upper panel, left). One molecule of non-toxin non-hemagglutinin (NTNHA) binds noncovalently to BoNT/A, consisting of light and heavy chains covalently linked by a disulfide bridge (yellow line), and protects it from destruction by digestive enzymes. At acidic pH, NTNHA also makes contact with the triskelion formed by a total of 12 hemagglutinins (HA) of three different sizes (HA17, HA33, and HA70), giving rise to the large progenitor toxin complex (stoichiometry in upper panel, right). Upon transition from the gut into tissue, the pH changes to neutral or slightly basic values, causing a conformational change in NTNHA that results in the release of BoNT/A and the dissociation from the relatively stable HA-triskelion (lower panel, left). Dissociation also takes place if solid BoNT/A formulations are reconstituted and injected into the tissue (not depicted). BoNT/A moves alone in tissue, lymph, and blood (lower panel, right) before it reaches its target, the terminal of peripheral cholinergic nerve cells (not shown here).

REFERENCES

1   https://www.plasticsurgery.org/documents/News/Statistics/2018/plastic-surgery-statistics-full-report-2018.pdf.
2   Pirazzini M, et al. Botulinum neurotoxins: Biology, pharmacology, and toxicology. *Pharmacol Rev.* 2017 Apr;69(2):200–235. doi:10.1124/pr.116.012658.
3   Amatsu S, et al. Multivalency effects of hemagglutinin component of type B botulinum neurotoxin complex on epithelial barrier disruption. *Microbiol Immunol.* 2018;62(2):80–89.
4   Lee K, et al. Molecular basis for disruption of E-cadherin adhesion by botulinum neurotoxin A complex. *Science.* 2014;344(6190):1405–1410.
5   Gu S, et al. Botulinum neurotoxin is shielded by NTNHA in an interlocked complex. *Science.* 2012;335(6071):977–981.
6   Amatsu S, et al. Crystal structure of Clostridium botulinum whole hemagglutinin reveals a huge triskelion-shaped molecular complex. *J Biol Chem.* 2013;288(49):35617–35625.
7   Kitamura M. Binding of botulinum neurotoxin to the synaptosome fraction of rat brain. *Naunyn Schmiedebergs Arch Pharmacol.* 1976;295(2):171–175.
8   Eisele KH, et al. Studies on the dissociation of botulinum neurotoxin type A complexes. *Toxicon.* 2011;57(4):555–565.
9   Heckly RJ, et al. On the size of the toxic particle passing the intestinal barrier in botulism. *J Exp Med.* 1960;111:745–759.
10 May AJ, et al. The absorption of Clostridium botulinum type A toxin from the alimentary canal. *Br J Exp Pathol.* 1958;39(3):307–316.

1 The Clinical Importance of Botulinum Toxin as an Injected Protein
Immunogenicity

Michael Martin

CONTENTS

The immunogenicity of BoNT/A is the ability of the antigen BoNT/A to induce an (adaptive) immune response, resulting in the production of antibodies specific for BoNT/A (Figure 1.1). Although not all antibodies arising to an antigen must necessarily be neutralizing, here the focus will be on neutralizing antibodies (nAbs) to BoNT/A as they are the clinically relevant ones.

INTRODUCTION – WHY NEUTRALIZING ANTIBODIES TO BoNT/A ARE AN ISSUE

BoNT/A is a very valuable pharma (pharmaceutical) protein that has been in use in neurology and in aesthetic medicine for nearly 30 years now. It has a very favorable drug profile with hardly any undesired pharmacological effects if administered properly. However, as with all pharma proteins in general, and especially with a bacterial protein like BoNT/A, the generation of neutralizing anti-drug antibodies (ADAs or nAbs) is an issue.

DOI: 10.1201/9781003008132-1

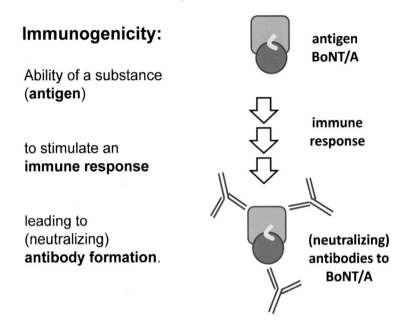

Immunogenicity:

Ability of a substance
(**antigen**)

antigen
BoNT/A

immune
response

to stimulate an
immune response

leading to
(neutralizing)
antibody formation.

(neutralizing)
antibodies to
BoNT/A

FIGURE 1.1 Definition of immunogenicity of BoNT/A.

Primary nonresponse means that a person already has nAbs to BoNT/A before the treatment starts and does not respond partially or fully. This is a rare event, possibly due to prior exposure to BoNT/A during food intoxication (a mild form of botulism).

Secondary nonresponse means that a patient responds very well to the BoNT/A treatment initially, but subsequently starts to produce nAbs and, over time, may become less responsive to the treatment (partial secondary nonresponder). In the worst cases, complete secondary nonresponse can occur if antibody titers are high enough to neutralize the drug completely (Figure 1.2). In clinical settings, this is a serious problem for the patient affected, as hardly any other treatment options remain. In aesthetic applications the consequences are less dramatic. Yet, the improvement in quality of life expected may not be achieved (anymore), resulting in frustration or even psychological problems.

Thus it is mandatory to deal with the issue of immunogenicity of BoNT/A and to discuss the immunological background leading to the generation of nAbs in order (1) to understand how the risk of antibody formation can be reduced and (2) to discuss what can be done to help a patient with antibody-dependent secondary therapy failure.

FREQUENCY OF nAbs TO BoNT/A IN PATIENTS

The first commercially available BoNT/A preparation ("Old Botox") induced the generation of nAbs in up to 17% of persons treated. More recent preparations of Botox® are much less immunogenic due to a change in the manufacturing procedure that resulted in a reduced load of pharmacologically inactive bacterial proteins, suggesting that these contributed to the immunogenicity of the drug. Frequencies published (Botox®, Dysport®, Xeomin® – data on other brands are not available) range between 0% and 3.5% over all indications (Fabbri et al. 2016; Bellows et al. 2019). In clinical indications, the problem of nAbs is more prominent most likely due to the higher doses of BoNT/A applied. Yet, especially in South East Asia, increasing doses of BoNT/A are now commonly used in relatively young persons in aesthetic uses (injections) as well. It is expected that frequencies of nAbs to BoNT/A will also increase in aesthetics.

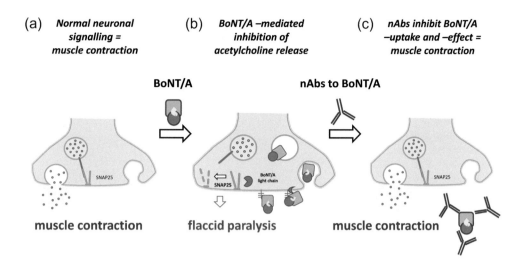

(a) *Normal neuronal signalling = muscle contraction*

(b) *BoNT/A –mediated inhibition of acetylcholine release*

(c) *nAbs inhibit BoNT/A –uptake and –effect = muscle contraction*

BoNT/A

nAbs to BoNT/A

muscle contraction   flaccid paralysis   muscle contraction

FIGURE 1.2   The consequence of neutralizing antibodies (nAbs) to BoNT/A at the neuro-muscular junction is lack of effectiveness = secondary nonresponsiveness. (a) SNAP25-mediated fusion of presynaptic vesicles with the plasma membrane results in release of neurotransmitter at the neuromuscular junction (MNJ). (b) BoNT/A is taken up into the nerve terminal and the light chain is translocated into the cytosol, where it cleaves and inactivates SNAP25. Vesicle fusion is inhibited and no acytelcholine is released, the result being a flaccid paralysis of innervated muscle. (c) Neutralizing antibodies to BoNT/A inhibit binding of the heavy chain to receptors. Thus, BoNT/A is not internalized and SNAP25 remains active, allowing vesicle fusion and neurotransmitter release. Innervated muscle contracts (again): no clinical BoNT/A effect.

IMMUNOGENICITY OF BoNT/A – REPEATED INJECTION OF BoNT/A RESEMBLES A VACCINATION

The repeated injection of the bacterial protein BoNT/A into a human being is reminiscent of a vaccination protocol. The success of a vaccination depends on a series of parameters, some of which are intrinsic to the person vaccinated, such as MHC (major histocompatibility complex, also called HLA) or immune status, while others can be influenced (by the physician), including dose and quality of antigen, and, most importantly, the presence of adjuvants (Table 1.1).

GENERAL CONSIDERATIONS ON THE IMMUNE REACTION OF A HUMAN BEING

The main task of the human immune system is to protect us from microbes, which are dangerous for us because they can multiply rapidly and either intoxicate us with their products (bacteria) or destroy the cells harboring and amplifying them (viruses). Therefore, the immune system has to decide quickly whether a full immune response, including the generation of antibodies, is required to fight the challenge or not. Our immune system uses the two criteria *dangerous* and *nonself* (= foreign) to decide if antibody production is necessary. These two decisions are made by two different types of leukocytes in a strictly hierarchical fashion. First, dendritic cells (DCs), sentinels of the innate arm of the immune system, recognize *danger signals* such as microbial surface molecules or microbial nucleic acids (Matzinger 2002). DCs become activated and mount a local acute inflammation with the aim being to contain and eliminate the microbes at the site of entrance. Activated DCs phagocytose what they have recognized as dangerous (the antigen), process it, and present peptides thereof in MHC class II molecules (antigen presentation) to the second decision maker. This is an antigen-specific T helper lymphocyte that recognizes presented *nonself* (= *foreign*) *peptides* and in turn also becomes activated. T cells finally help B lymphocytes to produce antibodies specific for

TABLE 1.1

Parameters Defining the Immunogenicity of a Vaccine

The success of a vaccination (formation of neutralizing antibodies) depends on:
- Individual parameters of the vaccinated person
  - HLA haplotype (Major histocompatibility complex (MHC) = the molecules that present peptide antigens)
  - immune status
- The composition of the antigen
- The dose of the antigen
- The presence of adjuvants
- The route of application

Possible additional contributions by
- Nonneutralizing anti-BoNT/A antibodies
- Crossreacting anti-Tetanus toxin antibodies

the dangerous antigen that initiated the whole process (Figure 1.3). Once produced in large quantities, antibodies support the fight against microbes by neutralizing them or their toxic products and/ or labeling them for subsequent destruction and removal by phagocytes.

THE IMMUNE REACTION OF A HUMAN BEING TO PURE BoNT/A

In order to decide if antibody production is an adequate response to the injection of pure bioactive BoNT/A, the immune system asks two questions in a strictly hierarchical fashion.

(1) Is pure bioactive BoNT/A *dangerous*?

And then, if (1) is answered with YES:

(2) Is BoNT/A *nonself (foreign)*?

This order is strictly fixed because DCs only phagocytose, process, and present antigen-derived peptides to T helper lymphocytes if they are optimally activated by a danger signal. If that is not guaranteed, no antigen presentation can take place, with the consequence that the adaptive immune system is not activated at all (Figure 1.4a).

The first question – *Is pure bioactive BoNT/A dangerous?* – translates into: Is BoNT/A a microbial surface structure that can activate DCs to become professional antigen-presenting cells? The answer is *no*. BoNT/A is not a surface protein of bacteria, therefore no receptors have evolved on DCs to recognize this intracellular protein. BoNT/A is not "classified" as a prototypical danger signal, thus by itself it is unable to activate DCs.

The second question – *Is BoNT/A nonself (foreign)?* – translates into: Can peptides derived from pure bioactive BoNT/A be presented and recognized as *nonself* by T helper lymphocytes? The answer is clearly *yes*. BoNT/A is a bacterial protein produced by *Clostridium botulinum*, and thus it is nonself or foreign. A recent study showed that BoNT/A-peptide specific T lymphocytes can be detected in a large number of patients treated with BoNT/A for neurological reasons (Oshima et al. 2011).

As the answer to the critical first question is *no*, DCs will not be activated to phagocytose BoNT/A or process and present peptides derived from the foreign bacterial protein to T helper cells. Thus, T cells will not be activated and, ultimately, antibodies to BoNT/A will not be produced. Pure and bioactive BoNT/A alone is a very weak immunogen as it lacks the mandatory microbial *danger signal* (Figure 1.4b).

But why then do some patients respond to BoNT/A treatment by producing nAbs?

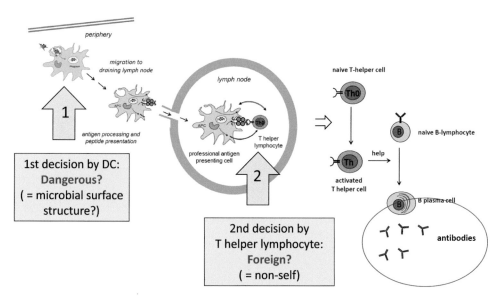

FIGURE 1.3 Scheme of the two-criteria two-step activation model of the human immune system leading to antibody production. (Left) Dendritic cells (DCs) act as sentinels and as first decision maker recognize microbial *danger signals*. DCs become activated and phagocytose the dangerous antigen, process it, and move to the draining lymph node (left). In the lymph node, they present peptides thereof in MHC class II molecules (antigen presentation) to the second decision maker, the naïve antigen-specific T helper lymphocyte (Tho) that recognizes presented *nonself (= foreign) peptides* and becomes activated (middle). T cells finally help B lymphocytes to produce antibodies specific to the dangerous antigen that initiated the whole process (right).

ADJUVANTS ENHANCE THE WEAK IMMUNE REACTION TO BoNT/A BY PROVIDING DANGER SIGNALS

The immunogenicity of a weak immunogen can be increased in a vaccine by adding adjuvants. Adjuvants provide the required danger signals lacking in weak immunogens like pure BoNT/A (Figure 1.5a). Intact killed bacteria or bacterial surface structures like flagellin are excellent adjuvants because they contain microbial surface structures. Adjuvants are mixed with the antigen and injected together at the same site. They activate DCs to phagocytose everything in their close vicinity, including the adjuvant and, most importantly, the weak immunogen, here BoNT/A. Being fully activated by the adjuvant, they digest the "co-phagocytosed" BoNT/A and present peptides thereof on MHC II to T helper lymphocytes, initiating a full adaptive immune response resulting in the production of antibodies to the weak immunogen (Figure 1.5b).

COMPONENTS IN BoNT/A PREPARATIONS THAT CAN ACT AS ADJUVANTS

All BoNT/A pharmaceuticals contain the 150kDa neurotoxin. Clostridia produce the neurotoxin in a large progenitor complex. The pharma protein BoNT/A is purified by different companies with different protocols to yield products with different degrees of purity (Frevert 2015).

COMPLEXING PROTEINS

Most brands contain bacterial complexing proteins. As of 2020, only two products free of complexing proteins are available: Xeomin® (Merz Pharmaceuticals, Germany), available worldwide; and

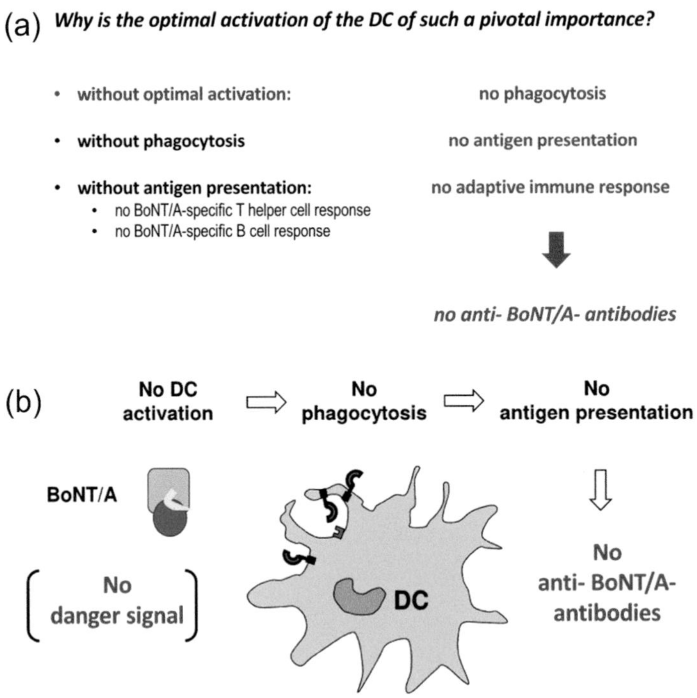

(a) *Why is the optimal activation of the DC of such a pivotal importance?*

- without optimal activation: no phagocytosis

- **without phagocytosis**   no antigen presentation

- **without antigen presentation:**   no adaptive immune response
  - no BoNT/A-specific T helper cell response
  - no BoNT/A-specific B cell response

no anti- BoNT/A- antibodies

(b)   **No DC   No   No
        activation ⟹ phagocytosis ⟹ antigen presentation**

BoNT/A

$$\left[\begin{array}{c}\text{No}\\ \text{danger signal}\end{array}\right]$$

DC

**No
anti- BoNT/A-
antibodies**

FIGURE 1.4 Optimal activation of dendritic cells is central to the immune response leading to antibody production. (a) Only optimally activated dendritic cells can serve as professional antigen presenting cells and initiate a full immune response. (b) Pure and bioactive botulinum neurotoxin A is unable to activate dendritic cells and to initiate an immune response because it lacks "danger signals".

Coretox® (Medytox, South Korea), available in South Korea. Apart from one protein (NTNHA), complexing proteins are hemagglutinins (HAs) by nature, with lectin-like moieties that bind to sugar residues contained in the surface glycoproteins of cells. By doing so they can crosslink receptors and activate immune cells, including DCs. In animals, HAs from *C. botulinum* increased the immunogenicity of BoNTs (Lee 2005; Kukreja 2009).

FLAGELLIN

C. botulinum employ flagella to move. Flagellin is contained in the fermentation product used as a starting material for purifying BoNT/A. If not completely removed (such as reported for Dysport® [Panjwani et al., 2008]), flagellin is a potent adjuvant capable of activating immune cells, including DCs, by binding to toll-like receptor 5 (Mizel et al. 2010).

DENATURED PROTEIN/PROTEIN AGGREGATES

BoNT/A can denature during the process of the production, purification, and pharmaceutical preparation of the drug, and during the reconstitution of solid formulations before use. The reasons for this can be exposure to heat, digestion by proteases, severe agitation, and very high salt concentrations during the preparation of the solid product. Denatured proteins tend to form protein aggregates. DCs recognize protein aggregates and are strongly activated. There is no dearth of literature on the immunogenicity of protein aggregates in biologicals (e.g. Rosenberg 2006).

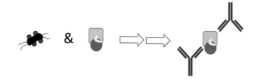

(a) **Adjuvants provide the "danger signal" missing in pure BoNT/A...**

...and neutralizing antibodies to BoNT/A can arise in patients.

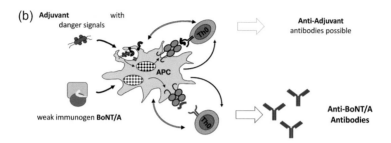

(b) **Adjuvant** with   **Anti-Adjuvant**
danger signals   antibodies possible

weak immunogen BoNT/A   **Anti-BoNT/A Antibodies**

FIGURE 1.5 Role of adjuvants in the immune response to BoNT/A. (a) The adjuvant provides the "danger signal" missing in pure bioactive BoNT/A. (b) Optimal activation of the dendritic cell by the adjuvant initiates phagocytosis of the weak immunogen BoNT/A, the processing to peptides, and the antigen presentation to naive T helper lymphocytes (Th0) specific to the peptide derived from BoNT/A ("blue" T helper cell). Subsequently, this allows B lymphocytes to produce anti-BoNT/A specific antibodies ("blue" antibodies). These can be neutralizing antibodies.

BACTERIAL DNA

It has been shown that some BoNT/A formulations are contaminated with bacterial DNA (Frevert et al. 2015). Microbial nucleic acids are potent danger signals and can be recognized by immune cells (via toll-like receptor 9) at extremely low concentrations.

Other factors possibly contributing to the immunogenicity of BoNT/A are summarized in Table 1.2.

MINIMIZING THE RISK OF ANTIBODY FORMATION IN PATIENTS TREATED WITH BoNT/A

In order to reduce the likelihood of antibody formation, it is mandatory to keep the amount of ingredients with adjuvant properties as low as possible in the drug formulation. Ideally, a product should only contain pure and bioactive BoNT/A without further bacterial ingredients. As additional bacterial proteins (complexing proteins or flagellin) are neither required for the pharmacological action on the nerve terminal nor for the stabilization of the pharma protein, they should be omitted. Furthermore, the utmost care should be taken during transport and storage, and while reconstituting for injection. All these different aspects may contribute alone or in combination to increase the immunogenicity of a BoNT/A pharmaceutical by providing "danger signals" for DCs. In summary, pure and bioactive BoNT/A without complexing proteins or other bacterial contaminants holds the lowest risk of antibody formation.

TABLE 1.2

Ingredients of Some BoNT/A Preparations That May Act as Adjuvant

- Bacterial cell wall components
- Flagellin
- Lectin-like components, such as hemagglutinins
- Protein aggregates, exposed hydrophobic amino acids in denatured protein
- Bacterial DNA

WHAT SHOULD BE DONE IF PATIENTS DEVELOP nAbs TO BoNT/A AND BECOME SECONDARY NONRESPONDERS?

Physicians have three options if patients become full secondary nonresponders:

- Stop treatment completely
- Discontinue treatment until nAbs have dropped below a clinically relevant level and then restart with a low-immunogenic BoNT/A preparation
- Continue treatment with a low-immunogenic BoNT/A

INTERRUPTION OF TREATMENT (TREATMENT HOLIDAY)

Studies have shown that one has to wait for several years before nAb titers drop to an undetectable level [Dressler & Bigalke 2002] probably due to the loss of antigen-specific long-lived B plasma and B memory cells. If treatment is restarted with the BoNT/A formulation that originally led to nAb formation, the immunological memory is activated and nAbs quickly reappear in most patients. However, if treatment is restarted with a low-immunogenic BoNT/A free of complexing proteins and other adjuvants, in some patients nABs may not reappear and treatment will again be successful (Dressler et al. 2018).

CONTINUATION OF TREATMENT WITH A BoNT/A PREPARATION WITH LOW IMMUNOGENICITY

In some patients who develop secondary therapy failure due to nAb formation, nAb titers may drop over time even if treatment is continued with a low immunogenic BoNT/A formulation (Hefter et al. 2012). A possible explanation is that the low-immunogenic BoNT/A formulation does not suffice to reactivate antigen-specific memory in these patients.

REFERENCES

Bellows S, et al. Immunogenicity associated with botulinum toxin treatment. *Toxins.* 2019 Aug 26;11(9). pii: E491. doi: 10.3390/toxins11090491.

Dressler D, et al. Botulinum toxin antibody type A titres after cessation of botulinum toxin therapy. *Mov Disord* 2002;17(1):170–173.

Dressler D, et al. Antibody-induced failure of botulinum toxin therapy: Re-start with low-antigenicity drugs offers a new treatment opportunity. *J Neural Transm* 2018;125(10):1481–1486.

Fabbri M, et al. Neutralizing antibody and botulinum toxin therapy: A systematic review and meta-analysis. *Neurotox Res* 2016;29(1):105–117.

Frevert J. Pharmaceutical, biological, and clinical properties of botulinum neurotoxin type A products. *Drugs R D* 2015;15(1):1–9.

Frevert J, et al. Presence of clostridial DNA in botulinum toxin products. *Toxicon* 2015;93(suppl.):S28–S41.

Hefter H, et al. Prospective analysis of neutralising antibody titres in secondary non-responders under continuous treatment with a botulinumtoxin type A preparation free of complexing proteins – a single cohort 4-year follow-up study. *BMJ Open* 2012;2(4). pii: e000646. doi: 10.1136/bmjopen-2011-000646.

Kukreja R, et al. Immunological characterization of the subunits of type A botulinum neurotoxin and different components of its associated proteins. *Toxicon* 2009;53(6):616–24.

Lee JC, et al. Production of anti-neurotoxin antibody is enhanced by two subcomponents, HA1 and HA3b, of Clostridium botulinum type B 16S toxin-haemagglutinin. *Microbiology* 2005;151(Pt 11):3739–3747.

Matzinger P. The danger model: A renewed sense of self. *Science* 2002;296(5566):301–305.

Mizel SB, et al. Flagellin as an adjuvant: Cellular mechanisms and potential. *J Immunol* 2010;185(10):5677–82.

Oshima M, et al. Human T-cell responses to botulinum neurotoxin. Responses in vitro of lymphocytes from patients with cervical dystonia and/or other movement disorders treated with BoNT/A or BoNT/B. *J Neuroimmunol* 2011;240–241:121–128.

Panjwani N, et al. Biochemical, functional and potency characteristics of type A botulinum toxin in clinical use. *Botulinum J* 2008;1:153–166.

Rosenberg AS. Effects of protein aggregates: An immunologic perspective. *AAPS J* 2006;8(3):E501–E507.

2 Optimizing Aesthetic Combination Treatments with Botulinum Toxin

Yates Yen-Yu Chao

CONTENTS

With the many advances in technology enabling us to intervene in the aging process and change tissue quality, increasing numbers of modalities of treatment are available and being given to patients who request antiaging procedures or further enhancement. As the morphological presentation of a living creature is composed of multiple layers of tissue, aging proceeds from inside out in multiple aspects, and so patients are usually approached and have to be treated by more modalities than just one. A combination of different treatments in one area starts as a trend and gradually becomes a must to achieve efficient and holistic effects. Patients often anticipate that these combinations will be performed in one visit since their problems are usually multiple, and these techniques have the reputation of being minimally invasive, easy, and simple. Botulinum toxin injection is one of the best known of these treatments and is often combined with other treatment modalities including device treatments, light-based procedures, and injectable products. There are even some novel practices that use toxins as one of the ingredients of a mixed formula. When the toxin is combined with other procedures, they could benefit from each other, adding synergic effects. However, they could also interfere with each other and cause adverse events.

COMBINATION SYNERGY AND CONCERNS

Botulinum toxin is indicated in aesthetic medicine mostly for mimetic muscle modulation (wrinkles and contours), muscle tone adjustment (refreshing and relaxing) and bulge reduction (contours), muscle rebalancing (facial landmark reposition and lifting), releasing tissue spaces, and smoothing the skin surface. The toxin is also used in superficial skin for skin quality enhancement and in vessels and skin appendages for function modulation.

DOI: 10.1201/9781003008132-2

ENERGY-BASED DEVICES

Energy-based devices usually deliver energy in a way that does not involve surface disruption. Energy input is transformed into heat, resulting in tissue damage to achieve treatment effects. However, the surface wounds of the skin do not interfere with the process of toxin administration and function apart from the destruction of tissue and subsequent swelling and protein coagulation. Dead tissue and denatured protein could be an adjuvant for arousing immune recognition. There is no literature documentation on the correlation, so it will require more studies and longer observation to ascertain what risk there may be in delivering toxin molecules in a tissue full of heat injury, but swelling and the breakdown of tissue dictate there may be more toxin spreading. For the procedures that have had local anesthetic tissue infiltration preparation, the tendency toward spreading could be increased further.

For clinical effects, the energy that shrinks or tightens tissues could be further augmented by the effect of toxin modulation with additional muscular contraction. Toxin intervention that trims the lower face curves through bulk relaxation or depressor inhibition could add more responses with earlier onset than the energy-related changes of the lower face and neck. Toxin-related muscle relaxation has long been misunderstood as the result of a "tightening injection" (which is what many patients request the toxin for). Tissue firming by heat destruction and tissue reconstruction, and facial landmark raising due to depressor muscle relaxation can reasonably be combined together.

When toxin imprecision or immunogenicity are the issues of concern, toxin injection and energy-based treatment could be separated into two areas (Figure 2.1a,b).

LIGHT-BASED DEVICES

Light-based treatments come in various different formats with varying extents of tissue injury. The consequences of light treatment can be altered tissue metabolic status, increased or decreased local circulation, heat damage, shockwave reactions and photochemical tissue injuries, structural destruction, cell death, protein coagulation, tissue desiccation, ablation, and different extents and formats of wounding. As with energy-based devices, toxins can be applied with concomitant light

(a)   (b)

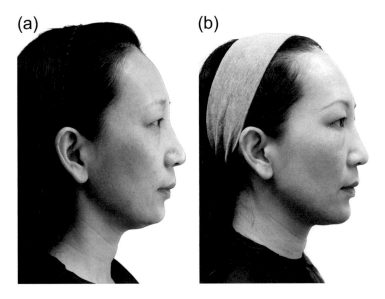

FIGURE 2.1   (a) Botulinum toxin A was administered in this patient following whole-face micro-focused ultrasound treatment on the same day. (b) Toxin modulation works well with energy lifting. The clinical improvement was satisfactory 1 month after the combined treatment.

treatments that would result in minimal tissue injury and surface wounds. Moderate to severe injury of the skin from light-based treatments raises more concern about the adjuvant denatured protein production and the possible immune arousal. The surface wounds and deep tissue injuries are minimal due to the fractionally delivered laser energy, but this damage can create tissue weakness and can change the pattern of toxin spread. Swelling of the tissue interferes with the extent and pattern of the toxin spreading as well.

However, the purposes of many light-based treatments are similar to those of botulinum toxin interventions: for example, the firming, tightening, and lifting of the skin is just like that achieved by energy-based devices and botulinum toxin; smoother and more radiant skin could be enhanced further by superficial toxin effects; the problem of redness and telangiectasia can be improved by toxins as well; and toxin injection has also been proved to be effective for scar management.

A toxin should be delivered after the healing of light treatment wounds. Same-day toxin treatment is more suitable for those light devices that make minimal tissue injuries or when toxin and light are delivered to different territories.

CHEMICAL PEELS

Botulinum toxin in practice is combined less often with chemical peels, but intradermal toxin injection has been reported to help to control acne and seborrhea, and also to enhance radiance and achieve a smoother texture. Those are also the goals of chemical peeling treatment.

INJECTABLE FILLERS

Being administered via a similar way of delivering process, filler injections are often combined with toxins.

Persistent trench-like wrinkles can be treated and filled with fillers; dynamic lines in the skin surface resulting from muscle squeezing could be released by the toxin. Facial shapes could be enhanced by volume augmentation through filler injection; part of the facial shape could be adjusted by the modulation of muscles with botulinum toxin. Fillers and toxin work synergistically like sculpting, aiming toward both volume reduction and augmentation.

Toxins are sometimes necessary to release tissue space in order to accommodate fillers; for example, the hypertonic mentalis muscle restricts the mental area, the tissue space required to accommodate fillers for chin augmentation. Filler facial recontouring can also benefit from the help of toxin muscle modulation. For example, filler distribution on the forehead could be more homogeneous if there are no contractions of the hyperactive frontalis muscle to disturb it (Figure 2.2a, b). The clinical effects of a line-tracing filler injection would last longer if these wrinkles could be controlled by toxin muscle relaxation (Figure 2.3a,b). Many problems related to filler placement could be less obvious if the activity of mimetic muscles could be damped in the vicinity of filler accumulation by a soft touch of botulinum toxin. For example, the structures of the medial cheek and the infraorbital region are highly mobile, with the elevation of stratified muscles including levator labi superioris, levator labi superioris alaequa nasi, zygomaticus major and minor, and so on. These mimetic muscles contract upon certain expressions and vocal functions that drag and pull the soft tissues. These forces bulge the soft tissue out and worsen the appearance of a poorly injected fullness. These contractions can clump the filled materials together, squeezing, distorting and dislocating these foreign substances (since these nonautologous gels connect only loosely to body tissue through weak affinity integration). Sometimes the overfilled superficial transparent gels can be grouped together and look like jelly pools. Light scattering magnifies these suboptimal works, which are often misnamed as the Tyndall effect. The bulging-out pressure under the excursion of elevator muscles reveals suboptimal unevenness, asymmetry, etc. Some of these filler problems become evident upon smiling or speaking, which embarrasses the patient. Similar problems occur also in the lateral orbit, near the zygomatic arch, overlying the malar ligaments, where mobility of

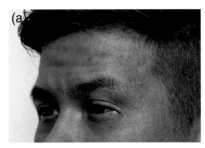
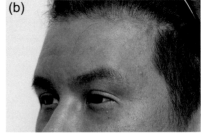

FIGURE 2.2 (a) Deep furrows, uneven surface, and suboptimal contour of the forehead were treated with hydrodissection-assisted filler augmentation and botulinum toxin frontalis modulation in one visit. The relaxation after toxin inhibition helps with the desired pattern of filler distribution. (b) Augmentation with dermal filler improved the wrinkles much more than the toxin effect alone.

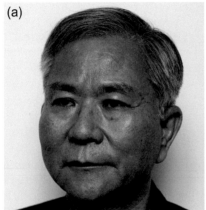
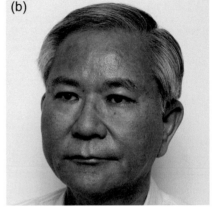

FIGURE 2.3 (a) The multiple aging wrinkles of this patient were treated with combined botulinum toxin and fillers. (b) The improvement of facial curves and removal of wrinkles were significant and looked natural.

the tissue is more prominent. Usually, minor imperfections in chin augmentation and cheek volume restoration could be detected more easily when muscles in the vicinity contract. In these situations, toxins could be gently applied to minimize muscle bulge and help to mask these faults (Figure 2.4a, b,c,d).

Conversely, toxin treatments also need the help of fillers to achieve better results. Masseter muscle toxin injection is often indicated for facial slimming or mandibular angle reduction. However, the bulging prominence of this corner tents up the cheek's soft-tissue envelope, masking the problem of underlying cheek hollowness. That is why hollowness appears in some patients when the mandibular angle diminishes after the masseter toxin treatment. Adjuvant filler volume restoration should be provided, and the reason behind the scenario should be explained in advance before the toxin treatment (Figure 2.5a,b). The Nefertiti lift, intended to improve the jawline by halting the downward traction of platysma fibers, should be accompanied with filler contouring around the mandibular margin to achieve better jawline defining effects.

Apart from interdependent works using toxin and fillers to achieve similar goals, the injections of toxin and fillers are usually required and carried out in one visit. Fillers are recommended to be applied first, then the toxin, if both agents are to be deposited in one day. The pattern of filler injection and the amount of fillers could have an impact on toxin spread. Fillers in tissue actually change the depth of muscle that toxin should target. The mode of needle insertion should be modified as well to

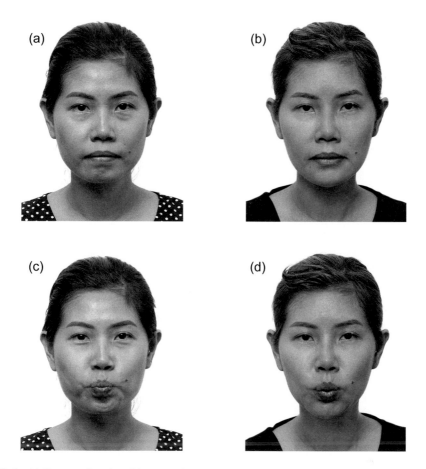

FIGURE 2.4 (a) Some patients' problems need more volume of filler to achieve satisfactory clinical effects. (b,c) The presence of filler underneath the skin and sometimes above muscles can be visible when muscles contract. (d) The use of minimal toxin in some highly mobile areas can reduce the effects of these structures and achieve a more elegant and natural result.

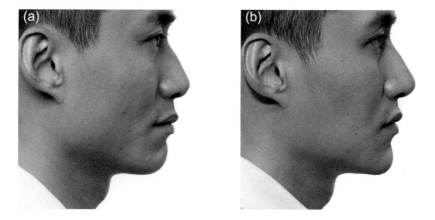

FIGURE 2.5 (a) Imbalance of volume distribution includes both excess and deficiency. A holistic approach to the problematic appearance corrects both deviations. Toxin to the masseter in this patient was combined with cheek filler modification and chin augmentation. (b) These treatments improved the profile proportion and smoothened the facial curve transition.

assure the delivery of toxin is correct in depth, ensuring an intramuscular injection. The presence of foreign substances – especially biostimulators – in the vicinity of the toxin injection would raise concerns about immune stimulation, either if the fillers had already been placed there or were just being injected together, as all the stimulations involve immune cells and inflammatory mediators.

COSMETIC SURGERY

Many aspects of cosmetic surgical procedures could benefit from the help of botulinum toxin. Toxin injection has been used for improving scar conditions. In the author's experience, it also helps the healing of wounds by inhibiting the contraction of neighboring muscles. Muscle contraction pulls the wounds where the skin and muscle connections through sutures are weak. Toxins have been found to have impacts on cultured fibroblast and have been used to control hypertrophy. Lip, nose, and eyelid surgeries could be further refined with toxins to achieve a better final presentation.

Toxins can be used for the preparation of surgical procedures in advance or for other nearby enhancement during the course of recovery, but preferably they should not be combined together on the same day, as they may confuse postoperative evaluation.

INTERFERENCE IN TOXIN COMBINATION

The wounding from lasers, peels, and surgeries and injuries from injections or energy-based treatments all could result in tissue edema and have impacts on toxin spread, increasing more treatment uncertainty. The alteration of layering relationship and thickness/depth of tissue can interfere with the judgment and precision of toxin administration and its efficacy in target tissues. Some treatments need special posttreatment care, like massages, that could also interfere with the distribution of toxins. Tissue dissection, injection tracts, the laser destruction plane, and the presence of foreign bodies predispose to unwanted preferential toxin spreading routes if the toxin is injected concomitantly or closely in time.

However, the toxin effect could be different in patients with altered muscle arrangements due to trauma or surgeries. The administered toxin could work contrarily against the goal of other treatments; for example, a dose on the forehead to suppress the elevation movement of frontalis could offset the clinical effects of energy-based lifting or surgical lifts. Asymmetry arising from concomitant toxin or surgery itself could complicate another symmetric treatment, since the first toxin administered could interfere with the initial assessment and posttreatment evaluation of the secondary one. Combination treatments could increase the complexity of the entire posttreatment evaluation. All these variable factors and impacts could possibly lead to a misdiagnosis and result in disputes between doctors and patients and between different medical service givers.

THE STRATEGY OF COMBINATION SEQUENCE

For surgical procedures, the use of botulinum toxin is preferably deferred until operative wounds have healed to avoid confusing evaluation before and after surgery.

For filler injections, the toxin could be combined in the same area and administered after the fillers. Toxin should be directed to the muscles and deposited as close as possible to the target fibers. For filling spaces that could be restricted or potentially disturbed by muscle contractions, toxins could be applied one or two weeks before to make room for the coming fillers.

For treatments combined with the use of energy-based devices, the toxin is better given as the last step or administered 1–2 weeks before the second treatment. For light-based treatments, the toxin can be applied at the same time as the lights or can be separated from light treatment by an interval of 1–2 weeks, especially when light treatments are more destructive or wounding in nature.

For multiple treatment combinations, the preferable sequence should be energy first, fillers second, then lights, and toxin last (Figure 2.6a,b,c,d,e).

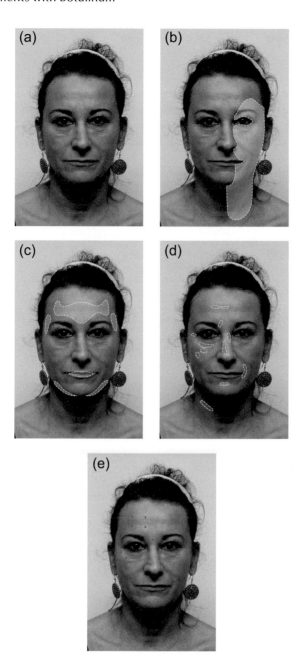

FIGURE 2.6 (a) Holistic aesthetic treatments involve a multimodality approach tackling different structural and morphological problems. (b) Energy-based tissue tightening should be applied first. (c) Fillers should first correct the large and deep volume problems, (d) and then the minor and superficial problems. (e) Toxin should be administered as the last step at different depths according to the treatment areas and indications.

MORE CONCERNS ABOUT TOXIN COMBINATIONS

More and more treatments emphasize biostimulation by means of foreign body tissue disruption, immune reaction, or low-grade tissue injury to achieve more self-tissue production. These components of tissue reaction include cytokines, inflammatory cells, collagen, elastin, vessels, and intercellular matrix. It has to be carefully observed if these stimuli from chemical substances, tissue damage, and foreign bodies lead to immune reaction through adjuvant protein aggregate, nucleic acid, and cell debris recognition or foreign antigen presentation when the pharmaceutical protein of botulinum toxin is administered concomitantly. As practice patterns become more diversified and toxin use is in the majority off-label, it looks as if the parameters indicated for this toxin molecule have become less restrictive. Toxins are being blended with various injectable materials as a cocktail ingredient. Similar behaviors have been claimed to be novel by mixing the toxin with autologous fat, PRP, and mixtures of mesotherapy. Though the cells and tissues are autologous, there are multiple punctures involved in meso-like treatments, and the processed tissues carry dead cells, tissue debris, contaminants, and pathogens.

BIBLIOGRAPHY

Carruthers J, et al. Consensus recommendations for combined aesthetic interventions in the face using botulinum toxin, fillers, and energy-based devices. *Dermatol Surg* 2016;42(5):586–597.

Chao YYY. Pan-Asian consensus-key recommendations for adapting the World Congress of Dermatology consensus on combination treatment with injectable fillers, toxins, and ultrasound devices in Asian patients. *J Clin Aesthet Dermatol* 2017;10(8):16–27.

Chao YYY. A single-visit approach using fillers and Incobotulinumtoxin A: Full face enhancement in Asian patients. *Plast Reconstr Surg Glob Open* 2018;6(10):e1909.

Farolch-Prats L. Facial contouring by using dermal fillers and botulinum toxin A: A practical approach. *Aesthetic Plast Surg* 2019;43(3):793–802.

Jeong TK. Mouth corner lift with botulinum toxin type A and hyaluronic acid filler. *Plast Reconstr Surg* 2020;145(3):538e–541e.

Zhu J, et al. The efficacy and safety of fractional CO_2 laser combined with topical type A botulinum toxin for facial rejuvenation: A randomized controlled split-face study. *Biomed Res Int* 2016;2016:3853754.

Zimbler M, et al. Update on the effect of botulinum toxin pretreatment on laser resurfacing results. *Arch Facial Plast Surg* 2012;14(3):156–158.

3 Antibody Formation and Botulinum Toxin Resistance

Jürgen Frevert and Yates Yen-Yu Chao

CONTENTS

IMMUNOLOGICAL CONCERNS

Jürgen Frevert

ANTIBODIES AGAINST BOTULINUM TOXIN

Botulinum neurotoxin and the complexing protein are bacterial proteins which can elicit the formation of antibodies (see Chapter 1). About 50% of patients treated in neurological indications develop antibodies against the complexing proteins (Goeschel et al. 1997). These antibodies do not play a role in the therapy; consequently, they do not affect the activity of the neurotoxin (Figure 3.1). In contrast, antibodies against the 150 kDa neurotoxin block the neurotoxin from binding (because not all Abs are neutralizing) and are therefore neutralizing antibodies and can lead to secondary nonresponse (resistance) (Figure 3.2). However, there are also antibodies that are directed against the neurotoxin but do not deactivate it. These antibodies are called nonneutralizing antibodies; they are probably directed against the functionally irrelevant epitopes of the neurotoxin. They are detected by a binding assay (immunoassay) whereas neutralizing antibodies are determined in an activity assay such as the mouse hemidiaphragma assay (Goeschel et al. 1997). An overview of different assays can be found in the article by Bellows and Jankovic (2019).

BnTX ANTIBODIES AND AESTHETIC PRACTICES

The development of antibodies against botulinum neurotoxin in aesthetic indication and secondary nonresponse has been a matter of controversy. It was claimed that the low doses applied in the treatment of facial wrinkles do not elicit the formation of antibodies, and that consequently the occurrence of secondary nonresponse would be negligible. However, the occurrence of antibodies is well documented in several publications (e.g. Borodic et al. 2007, Dressler et al. 2010, Torres et al. 2014, Stephan et al. 2014). Because of substantially higher doses of the antigen (150 kDa neurotoxin), the development of neutralizing antibodies is more common in therapeutic indications. In clinical studies (glabellar lines). the rate of antibody formation is reported to be below 1% (Fabbri et al. 2016), which is not unexpected because the duration of the studies is usually short (<2 years). The occurrence of treatment resistance is well known in numerous practices but currently there are

DOI: 10.1201/9781003008132-3

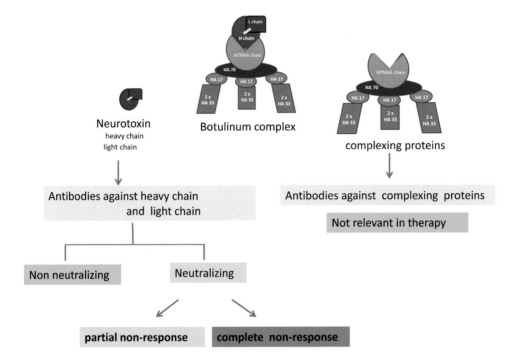

FIGURE 3.1 Development of antibodies against botulinum toxin proteins in the therapy with botulinum toxin.

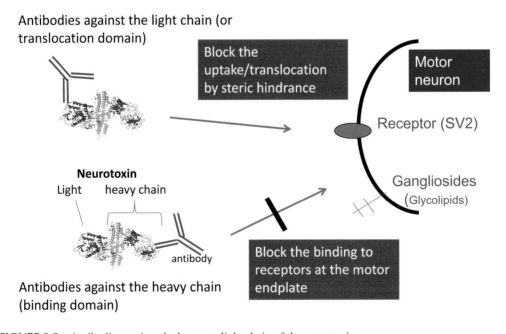

FIGURE 3.2 Antibodies against the heavy or light chain of the neurotoxin.

no published numbers. In contrast to therapeutic indications where patients are usually treated over a long period of time in the same clinic, patients with aesthetic indications switch practices or stop treatment because they feel no benefit from the treatment (possibly because of antibody development). Physicians in the aesthetic field are also not as aware of secondary nonresponse as physicians in the therapeutic field. Therefore, it is difficult to make any conclusive statement about the prevalence of antibodies against botulinum neurotoxin in aesthetic indications.

WHEN RESISTANCE DEVELOPS

The formation of antibodies is a continuous process, starting with a low antibody titer without clinical consequences; this is followed by higher titers, which can partially prevent the effect of the injection (*partial nonresponse*); and finally by a complete neutralization (*complete nonresponse*) in cases where a high titer is formed so that all neurotoxin molecules are captured by antibodies (Dressler 2000, Dressler & Bigalke 2017) (Figure 3.3). Antibody titers required to cause nonresponse (resistance) to botulinum toxin have not been defined, and immune responses can differ between treatment resistant patients (Dressler et al. 2010).

Patients treated repeatedly show a tendency to require a lower dose or show a longer duration of effect, probably because of muscle atrophy or a reduced number of neurotoxin targets (Small 2014). The formation of an antibody titer can usually be observed when the injected dose does not show the same effect as at the beginning of the therapy and does not result in a similar duration. Consequently, a higher dose is injected to achieve the same effect and duration ("dose creep"). This was corroborated in a recent study reporting that patients with an antibody titer who still respond require a higher dose (Hefter et al. 2019). A higher dose can compensate for low or intermediate antibody titers, as has been shown in neurological indications (Dressler et al. 2002).

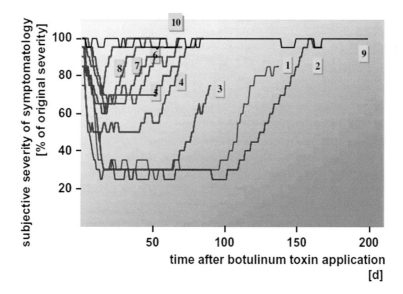

FIGURE 3.3 Development of secondary nonresponse in a patient treated with botulinum toxin. (From Dressler & Bigalke 2017, with permission.)

However, this would initiate a vicious cycle because a higher amount of antigen (neurotoxin) would further increase the antibody formation so that an even higher dose is required, which further drive antibody development. If the treatment is terminated, the antibody titer decreases over time because plasma cells, which produce the antibodies and memory B cells, disappear. This allows the physician – when the titer is low enough – to reinitialize treatment with a low immunogenicity product. However, the reduction of the antibody titer is not always guaranteed: after the cessation of treatment in 13 patients (cervical dystonia) with complete treatment failure, 8 of the patients showed a decrease after 750 days whereas 5 of the patients did not show any drop in the titer after 1,500 days (Dressler & Bigalke 2002). This demonstrates marked individual differences in the reduction of the titers. It was demonstrated that treatment with a low immunogenicity product after development of resistance is possible after some time: a patient (violinist) with hand cramp who developed secondary nonresponse after long-term treatment with onabotulinumtoxin was treated successfully with incobotulinumtoxin after 18 months of not being injected with onabotulinumtoxin (Ramos et al. 2014).

There is no general rule as to how long the "treatment holiday" should last before the patient becomes responsive again, but a period of at least 2 years would be required. The time is dependent on the height of the titer developed by the patient and – as mentioned above – on the individual kinetics of the antibody decrease.

Are there differences in the immunogenicity of the products? As described in detail in Chapter 1 on immunogenicity, the immune system, especially dendritic cells, must be activated to initiate the development of antibodies. Onabotulinumtoxin, abobotulinumtoxin, and prabotulinumtoxin contain proteins (complexing proteins and flagellin in abobotulinumtoxin) and inactive neurotoxin which can activate the immune system; they act as adjuvants, whereas incobotulinumtoxin contains only the active neurotoxin. Consequently, the immunogenicity of incobotulinumtoxin is very low. Indeed, so far, a secondary nonresponse induced by incobotulinumtoxin has not been reported in treatment naïve patients. The low immunogenicity of incobotulinumtoxin was also demonstrated in a study with therapeutic indications: patients who developed an antibody titer and partial secondary nonresponse were treated with a relatively high dose (200 U of incobotulinumtoxin) every 3 months for 4 years. Another cohort with an antibody titer was left untreated. As expected, the mean antibody titer decreased. Surprisingly, the mean antibody titer in the treated cohort decreased in a similar fashion (Hefter et al. 2012). In a long-term trial with patients suffering from neurological disorders, the low immunogenicity could be confirmed: so far, not a single patient had developed antibodies after treatment with incobotulinumtoxin (Hefter et al. 2020). In the first study that reports data for the prevalence of antibodies in different neurological indications, it was calculated that the prevalence of antibody formation in 596 patients was 13.9% at a treatment duration of 5.6 years (Albrecht et al. 2019). This prevalence represents a substantially higher number than the number reported before for therapeutic indication (e.g. Lacroiz-Demazes et al. 2017: 3.6%). It was found that 6% of the patients treated with abobotulinumtoxin and 7% treated with onabotulinumtoxin developed antibodies (Albrecht et al. 2019). It can be concluded that the antibody formation in aesthetic indications is also markedly higher than the low numbers published previously. However, there is no similar study available analyzing antibody formation over a long treatment period.

In summary: to avoid the formation of antibodies and the development of resistance, it is recommended that a low immunogenicity product is used with the smallest dose that achieves the desired clinical effect, and the injection interval should be as long as possible. If a patient has developed resistance, treatment could be reinitiated after a break of 1–2 years (without any guarantee of success).

CLINICAL OBSERVATION OF BOTULINUM TOXIN
RESISTANCE IN AESTHETIC PRACTICES

Yates Yen-Yu Chao

The possibility of antibody formation and botulinum toxin resistance is generally believed to be low in aesthetic practice – or rather, most practitioners judge the chances of antibody formation in treatment using botulinum toxin in aesthetic practice on the basis of their own clinical impressions. However, only the neutralizing antibodies against botulinum toxin would interfere with the clinical effects of the toxin and be felt through clinical observation. The actual prevalence of antitoxin antibodies in patients who have received botulinum toxin injections is much higher. And even with the neutralizing antibody, the rate of its detectable existence by laboratory examinations is not equal to the rate of clinically noticeable symptoms. In my experience, the early signs of clinical resistance are extremely mild and could be easily missed.

Though the dosing of the toxin for aesthetic treatment is generally low compared with therapeutic indications, with more and more novel applications for aesthetic purposes (especially the emerging uses on the body), the collective toxin units from multifocal administration in a single patient have been far more than the doses used before. With the many usages of toxin (not just for wrinkles), patients now start their aesthetic treatment journey and have their toxin much earlier than before, at a younger age. With the growing tendency to use combinations with toxin injections and other wounding procedures or the concomitant administration with injectable or implantable foreign substances, there should be growing concerns about potential immunogenicity. The dermal deployment of toxin should be watched more closely because of its closeness to a denser population of antigen-presenting cells there. All these evolutions of practice encourage us to take the issue of toxin resistance seriously, even if the toxin is just for aesthetic purposes.

Initial symptoms of toxin resistance include decreased clinical efficacy, incomplete clinical effects, or shortened longevity. These presentations are just the different facets of one story. Decreased efficacy could often be detected by generalized or focal remaining muscle activity or incomplete muscle block after the onset time. More residual muscle activity at a certain time could be considered as shortened longevity. As more and more practices now refine their treatments with less overwhelming freezing, the detection of subtle insufficiency needs more careful and vigilant observation, especially the early effects 1–2 weeks after treatment. However, toxin treatments have been too routine. Returning checks are often omitted and considered unnecessary. Compared with the smaller areas of the lateral corners of orbicularis oculi or glabella muscles, the broad forehead muscle reflects these decreases in efficacy more sensitively.

In one of our studies using the recombinant receptor-binding domain (RBD) via an E. coli expression system as the substrate, to test the existence of antibodies in patients' serum against the specific epitope (RBD) of the heavy chain (unpublished study), different patients with moderate to severe clinical symptoms of botulinum toxin resistance and complete treatment failure were recruited and tested using indirect ELISA (Figure 3.4). Signals of the exams positively correlate with the clinical severity of loss of toxin effects. Serum specimens from some of these patients were also sent for mouse diaphragm assay (MDA). The clinical complete failure case that was strongly positive in the RBD ELISA test was tested as half positive by MDA. The other cases with mild to moderate ELISA signals were all examined as negative by MDA.

The antibody against RBD is one of the many different neutralizing Abs that could interfere with clinical toxin effects. However, the mouse assay that is generally considered as the standard method of detecting toxin resistance might not be sensitive enough to detect early resistant cases.

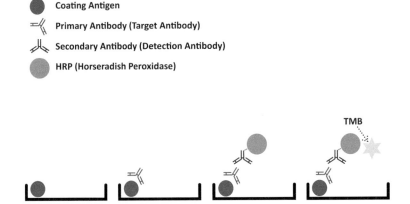

● Coating Antigen

Primary Antibody (Target Antibody)

Secondary Antibody (Detection Antibody)

● HRP (Horseradish Peroxidase)

FIGURE 3.4 Indirect ELISA was designed using recombinant peptide fragments corresponding to the receptor-binding domain of the toxin heavy chain of the serotype A of botulinum toxin as the coating antigen. The signal level of the test reflects the amount of the specific antibody binding to this epitope.

REFERENCES

Albrecht P, et al. High prevalence of neutralizing antibodies after long-term botulinum neurotoxin therapy. *Neurology* 2019;92:1–7.

Bellows S, et al. Immunogenicity associated with botulinum toxin treatment. *Toxins* 2019;11:491 pii: E491. doi:10.3390/toxins11090491

Borodic G. Botulinum toxin, immunologic considerations with long-term repeated use, with emphasis on cosmetic applications. *Facial Plast Surg Clin North Am.* 2007;1:11–16.

Dressler D. *Botulinum Toxin Therapy.* Stuttgart, New York:Thieme Verlag; 2000.

Dressler D, et al. Antibody induced botulinum toxin therapy failure: Can it be overcome by increased botulinum toxin doses? *Eur Neurol* 2002;47:118–121.

Dressler D, et al. Antibody induced failure of botulinum toxin a therapy in cosmetic indications. *Dermatol Surg* 2010;36(suppl 4):2182–2187.

Dressler D, Bigalke H. Immunological aspects of botulinum toxin therapy. *Expert Rev Neurother.* 2017;17(5):487–494.

Fabbri M, et al. Neutralizing antibody and botulinum toxin therapy: A systematic review and meta-analysis. *Neurotox Res* 2016;29(1):105–117.

Göschel H, et al. Botulinum A toxin therapy: Neutralizing and nonneutralizing antibodies – therapeutic consequences. *Exp Neurol* 1997;147:96–102.

Hefter H, et al. Prospective analysis of neutralising antibody titres in secondary non-responders under continuous treatment with a botulinumtoxin type A preparation free of complexing proteins – a single cohort 4-year follow-up study. *BMJ Open* 2012;4;2(4). pii: e000646. doi: 10.1136/bmjopen-2011-000646

Hefter H, Rosenthal D, Bigalke H, Moll M. Clinical relevance of neutralizing antibodies in botulinum toxin long-term treated still-responding patients with cervical dystonia. *Ther Adv Neurol Disord.* 2019 Dec 16;12:1756286419892078. doi: 10.1177/1756286419892078.

Hefter H, et al. Effective long-term treatment with incobotulinumtoxin (Xeomin®) without neutralizing antibody induction: A monocentric, cross-sectional study. *J Neurol* 2020. doi: 10.1007/s00415-019-09681-7

Lacroix-Desmazes S, Mouly S, Popoff MR, Colosimo C. Systematic analysis of botulinum neurotoxin. Type A immunogenicity in clinical studies. *Basal Ganglia* 2017; 9:12–17.

Ramos, et al. Clinical response to Incobotulinumtoxin A, after demonstrated loss of clinical response to Onabotulinumtoxin A and Rimabotulininumtoxin B in a patient with musician's dystonia. *Mov Disord Clin Pract.* 2014;1(4):383–385.

Small R. Botulinum toxin injection for facial wrinkles. *Am Fam Physician* 2014;90(3):168–175.

Stephan F, et al. Clinical resistance to three types of botulinum toxin type A in aesthetic medicine. *J Cosmet Dermatol* 2014;13(4):346–348.

Torres S, et al. Neutralizing antibodies to botulinum neurotoxin type A in aesthetic medicine: Five case reports. *Clin Cosmet Investig Dermatol* 2014;7:11–17.

4 Conversion and Calculations between Different Commercial Toxin Products

Jürgen Frevert and Yates Yen-Yu Chao

CONTENTS

TECHNICAL CONSIDERATIONS

Jürgen Frevert

MANUFACTURE OF BoNT PRODUCTS

The manufacturing process of botulinum toxin products approved in aesthetic indication starts with the fermentation of *Clostridium botulinum* type A. The so called Hall strain of *Clostridia botulinum* type A is employed by the manufacturers (see Table 4.1), although Allergan's strain Hall-hyper, which might have different sporulation properties (Bradshaw et al. 2004), seems to be different. Although it is not clear whether the strains are the same, the amino acid sequence of the neurotoxin in all products seems to be identical (Dineen et al. 2003). In essence, the pharmacologically active substance – the 150 kDa neurotoxin – in all products acts identically, which is reflected in similar clinical properties. However, this does not mean that the neurotoxin in all products is completely identical because the manufacturing process of the products is different; biotechnologists have coined the phrase "the product is the process" because the tertiary structure (folding) of the protein might be affected by the purification process (Schellekens and Casadevall 2004). One can speculate that this could lead to a different epitope structure, implying that antibodies formed against one product might not bind to all epitopes of another product.

    After growth and lysis of the clostridia, the neurotoxin is purified by applying different purification protocols (Figure 4.1): onabotulinumtoxin is purified by precipitation with ethanol, followed by a series of ammonium sulphate precipitation, and dissolution ("crystallization") resulting in a large complex (900 kDa complex) (Schantz & Johnson 1992) composed of the 150kDa neurotoxin attached to several other proteins, the so-called complexing proteins or neurotoxin associated proteins (NAPs). Abobotulinumtoxin A is processed by applying ion exchange chromatography (Panjwani et al. 2008), providing a mixture of complexes whose identity is not published by the

TABLE 4.1

Comparison of Leading Botulinum Toxin-A Products

Botulinum toxin type A	AbobotulinumtoxinA	OnabotulinumtoxinA	IncobotulinumtoxinA
Brand names	Dysport®	Botox®,	Xeomin®,
Clostridial strain	Hall	Hall-hyper	ATCC3502 (Hall)
Presentation	Freeze-dried (lyophilized) powder for reconstitution	Vacuum-dried powder for reconstitution	Freeze-dried (lyophilized) powder for reconstitution
Isolation process	Precipitation and chromatography	Precipitation	Precipitation and chromatography
Composition	*Clostridium botulinum* type A neurotoxin HA and non-HA protein Flagellin	*Clostridium botulinum* type A neurotoxin HA and non-HA protein	*Clostridium botulinum* type A neurotoxin
Excipients	500 U vial‡: 125 μg human serum albumin 2.5 mg lactose	100 U vial‡: 0.5 mg human serum albumin 0.9 mg NaCl	100 U vial‡: 1 mg human serum albumin 4.6 mg sucrose
Molecular weight (kD)	Not published	900	150
Approximate total clostridial protein content‡	4.35 ng (500 U)	5.0 ng (100 U)	0.44 ng (100 U)
Neurotoxin protein load (neurotoxin per 100 U‡)	0.65 ng	0.73 ng	0.44 ng
Specific neurotoxin potency (Potency per ng neurotoxin)	154 U/ng	137 U/ng	227 U/ng

Source: Modified from Frevert 2015.

‡ Units of measurement for the three commercially available BoNT/A preparations are proprietary to each manufacturer and are not interchangeable.

*Depending on the number of units. HA, hemagglutinin.

manufacturer. In addition, aboboutulinumtoxin contains an additional bacterial protein (not a complexing protein), flagellin (see Chapter 3 on immunogenicity). On the other hand, incobotu-linumtoxin is purified in a series of chromatographic steps, resulting in a pure 150 kDa neurotoxin without any other clostridial proteins or other impurities such as nucleic acids, which are found in onabotulinumtoxin (Groenewald & Frevert 2015). The complexing proteins are unnecessary for the therapeutic effect, as they do not influence the biological activity. In addition, they do not have any benefit for the pharmaceutical properties of the products (Frevert & Dressler 2010).

MEASURING THE BIOLOGICAL ACTIVITY

All batches of BoNT products are tested for potency before release. The assay must be able to quantify the amount of active molecules of the 150 kDa neurotoxin, i.e., all the steps of the mode of action must be captured (see Chapter 1 on pharmacology for the mechanism of action). The assay approved for all products by all health agencies was the LD50 assay, an assay developed in toxicology to quantify the toxicity of chemicals (Zbinden et al. 1981) (Figure 4.2). In this assay, 0.5 mL of a

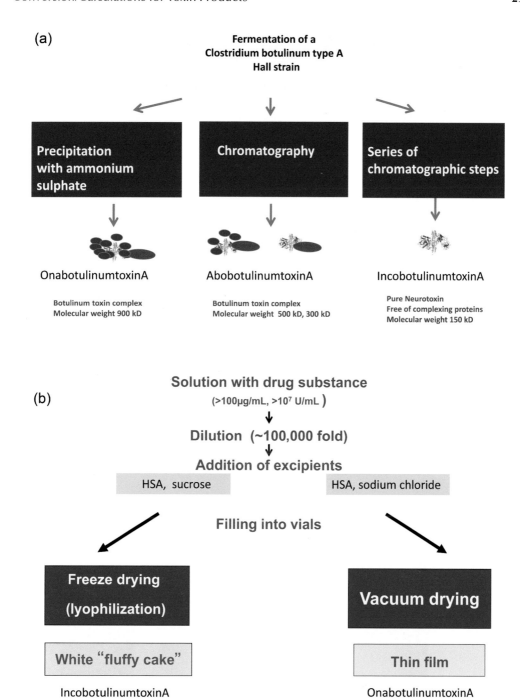

FIGURE 4.1 Manufacturing of botulinum toxin products. A. Manufacturing the drug substance (solution with neurotoxin or neurotoxin embedded in complex). B. Manufacturing of drug product (Onabotulinumtoxin, Icobotulinumtoxin).

series of different dilutions of botulinum toxin are injected i.p. into groups of mice. After 72 hours, the number of dead mice is counted. This allows the calculation of the LD50 unit, which is defined as the dose lethal to 50% number of mice in each group. The assay is conducted in parallel with a standard proprietary to every company, and the potency is calculated in comparison with the standard ("parallel line assay"). Because several parameters in this biological assay differ from company to company (animal-related differences, e.g. strain, age, diet, caging), most importantly the diluent and the standard, the results of the LD50 assay can differ. Consequently, the LD50 units are proprietary for each product and cannot be compared directly, which underscores the need for clinical head-to-head studies (Figure 4.3). For the measurement of onabotulinumtoxin, the reconstituted vial is further diluted about 100-fold with saline (Hunt & Clarke 2009). Abobotulinumtoxin is analyzed in a solution containing gelatin and phosphate buffer (Hambleton & Pickett 1994), whereas incobotulinumtoxin is diluted in saline containing human serum albumin (Dressler et al. 2012).

Recently, the LD50 assay has been replaced by a cell-based assay (CBA). The potency of onabotulinumtoxin is determined in human neuroblastoma cells (Fernandez-Salas et al. 2012). Induced pluripotent stem cells (iPSC) are applied to analyze the potency of incobotulinumtoxin (Whitemarsh et al. 2012) (Figure 4.4). The details of the CBA for abobotulinumtoxin have not yet been published. The CBAs are extensively crossvalidated with the LD50 assay to provide the same potency result (the units are still LD50 units, analyzed with a different procedure).

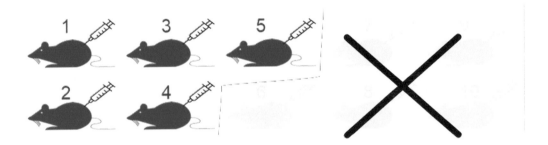

FIGURE 4.2 Potency testing of every batch of a botulinum toxin product is performed before batch release – ensuring consistent potency. Previously, the LD50 test was used with mice (1 LD50 unit = the amount of neurotoxin that kills 50% of a group of mice).

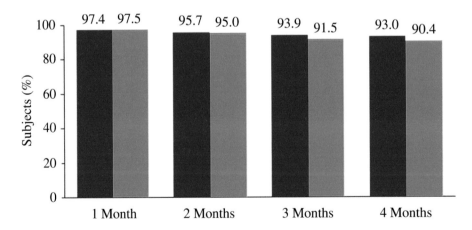

FIGURE 4.3 Head-to-head trial of incobotulinumA (left columns) and onabotulinumtoxinA (right columns) in the treatment of glabellar lines: proportion of subjects (n = 255) satisfied with treatment. (From Kane MA, et al. *Dermatol Surg.* 2015, 41(11):1310-9, with permission.)

The protease activity of the light chain can also be determined with specific assays. However, these assays only capture a part of the activity (binding and translocation are not analyzed). Therefore, it is not adequate to draw conclusions from only light chain measurements as has been reported in the literature (Field et al. 2018). The authors found a higher protease activity in abobotulinumtoxin and concluded that it has a higher amount of active BoNT/A molecules, resulting in a longer duration of action when injected in an equivalent dose compared to the other products. But only the determination of all steps of the mode of action (binding, translocation, and cleavage of SNAP25) would allow a conclusion on the amount of active molecules in abobotulinumtoxin.

COMPARISON OF BOTULINUM PRODUCTS IN POTENCY ASSAYS

Onabotulinumtoxin and incobotulinumtoxin were compared in the Allergan LD50 assay; the potency of incobotulinumtoxin in this assay was 25% lower (Hunt & Clarke 2009). An analysis with the Merz LD50 assay showed that onabotulinumtoxin and incobotulinumtoxin were equipotent (Dressler et al. 2012). This discrepancy can be explained (partly) by the different diluents. In the Allergan assay, the reconstituted vial is diluted with saline only, which leads to a low concentration of HSA <5µg/mL – very different from the concentration in the clinic, where the concentration is between 100 ng/mL and 200 ng/mL for onabotulinumtoxin and incobotulinumtoxin. It is known from pharmacological studies that a "protein stabilizer" (like HSA or gelatin) or a surfactant are necessary to keep the BoNT molecules in solution when the concentration is extremely low (pg/mL). The function of such a stabilizer is not exactly known; it was speculated that it prevents the neurotoxin from sticking to the glass surface of the vial (Kutschenko et al. 2019). In contrast to the Allergan assay, HSA is added to the saline to assay incobotulinmtoxin to mimic the reconstituted vial in the clinic. Because the diluent in the assay reflects the condition in the clinic, one can draw the conclusion that onabobotulinumtoxin is equipotent to incobotulinumtoxin. This is confirmed in another potency assay, the mouse hemi-diaphragma assay (Bigalke & Rummel 2015). In this assay, the biological activity is determined ex vivo in an organ bath with a Nervus phrenicushemi-diaphragma tissue (mouse). There was a slightly lower activity of onabobotulinum in this assay when compared with incobotulinumtoxin (Pan et al. 2019). No study of the products in a cell-based assay has been published, probably because the different excipients in the product would affect the

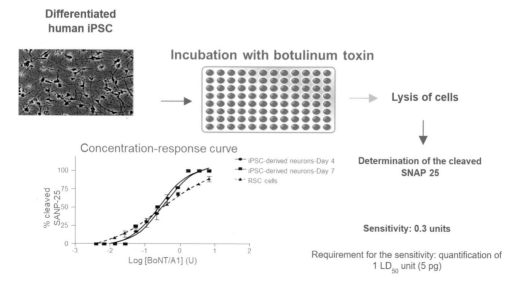

FIGURE 4.4 The current highly sensitive cell-based assay.

assay, which prevents a direct comparison. In summary, preclinical assays demonstrate a 1:1 dose relationship of onabotulinumtoxin:incobotulinumtoxin.

In contrast to the potency equivalence, the dose ratio between onabotulinumtoxin (or incobotulinumtoxin) and abobotulinumtoxin is not clear. In an early study, onabotulinumtoxin and abobotulinumtoxin were analyzed with the Allergan assay and with the Ipsen LD50 assay. In contrast to the Allergan assay, the Ipsen assay (or the Speywood assay, named after one of the companies who distributed Dysport) uses a diluent containing gelatin as a stabilizer (a proxy of HSA in the products) in a phosphate buffer. A standard preparation of abobotulinumtoxin (500 U) compared with 100 onabotulinumtoxin showed in this potency assay a ratio of 1:1.7 (Hambleton 1994). Other studies report a dose ratio of 1:2.86 (Van den Bergh & Lison 1996) and 1:1.9 (First et al. 1994). These results cannot be easily translated into clinical efficacy because the amount of HSA in a vial of abobotulinumtoxin is relatively low compared to the other products. If 500 U abobotulinumtoxin are reconstituted with 2.5 mL saline, the concentration of HSA would be only 50 µg/mL (onabobotulinumtoxin 200µg/mL, incobotulinumtoxin 400µg/mL). It was demonstrated recently that the concentration of HSA affects the amount of active BoNT/A detectable in the hemi-diaphragma assay (Kutschenko et al. 2019). The authors concluded that the "low content of HSA is also accountable for the required higher dose of abobotulinumtoxin compared to the doses of the other two BoNT/A products that contain HSA in higher concentrations". Further, they report that there was a time-dependent loss of activity at low concentrations of HSA (like in abobotulinumtoxin). This might explain that different dose ratios are reported in the literature for preclinical assays and in clinical studies (see below). Consequently, only clinical head-to-head studies can provide an adequate dose relationship for abobotulinumtoxin to the other products.

Amount of Neurotoxin Protein in and Specific Potency of BoNT/A1 Products

The respective amounts of the 150 kDa neurotoxin per 100 U were 0.73 ng for onabotulinumtoxin, 0.65 ng for abobotulinumtoxin, and 0.44 ng for incobotulinumtoxin (Frevert 2010) (Table 4.1). It has to be stressed that the amount of protein does not provide any information about the content of active neurotoxin molecules, which can only be determined in an activity/potency assay. From these data, the specific potency or biological activity (U) per mass of neurotoxin protein was calculated giving incobotulinumtoxin the highest specific biological activity (U/ng neurotoxin) at 227 U/ng compared with 137 U/ng for onabotulinumtoxin and 154 U/ng for abobotulinumtoxin (although the units of abobotulinumtoxin are different, as described for abobotulinumtoxin). Because the 0.73 ng of onabotulinum have a similar potency as incobotulinumtoxin, it is hypothesized that that part of the neurotoxin in onabotulinumtoxin may be inactive or denatured due to the specific vacuum-drying process used in the manufacture of the final drug (Frevert 2010, Goodnough & Johnson 1992). The injection of a higher amount of antigenic protein (neurotoxin) which is partly denatured might have immunogenic consequences (see Chapter 3 on immunogenicity).

DIFFERENT BOTULINUM TOXIN A PRODUCTS IN AESTHETIC PRACTICES

Yates Yen-Yu Chao

Theoretically, when the same amount of active botulinum toxin molecules from different products are injected into subjects in the same way, the clinical efficacy and longevity should be the same. However, the claims that the different commercially available products are the same – or are different – might not be reliable. Results from different institutions appear severely discrepant. Of course, conditions can differ from one laboratory to another; nevertheless, the ratio between different kits in practical clinical settings, i.e., in normal human physical status, is what the practitioners really care about. Any thesis based on laboratory assays has to be further examined by clinical studies. However, even the interpretations and initiatives could deviate as well and be biased.

CLINICAL STUDIES ON THE COMPARISON OF BOTULINUM TOXIN A PRODUCTS

A 12-month retrospective multicenter study of 1,256 patients being treated for the upper face with switches found no difference between INCO and ONA in terms of patient satisfaction, dosage, and tolerance (Prager et al. 2012). Another 4-month prospective multicenter double-blind study on 381 cases of glabellar frown lines found INCO and ONA equal in terms of onset time, clinical efficacy, and patient satisfaction (Sattler et al. 2010). The treatment dose was lowered (from 24 to 20 U). Injectors were blinded to the products that were used. Kane et al. (2015) repeating the study in 2015, proved the two toxins to be generally equal in potency on 250 female patients. The split-face study by Muti for crow's feet with lower doses (12U) of INCO and ONA and crossing over found them almost the same in clinical efficacy, functioning time, and patient satisfaction. The Moers-Carpi (2012) study with INCO 30 U compared with ONA 20 U was based on an unfair preset assumption (because overfilling a muscle unit does not result in additional measurable effect) that led to a biased conclusion of an efficiency ratio of 3:2 (Ona to Inco). This conclusion was then matched in reverse by a split-face study of ONA 12U and Inco 8U for frown lines that concluded the opposite (a ratio of 2:3) (Prager et al. 2017). Most of the meta-analysis on the comparison between INCO and ONA in aesthetic uses concluded their similar clinical efficacy without much difference.

The ratio between ABO and ONA has long been debated. The problem of overdosing existed in earlier studies. The diffusion issue and injection pattern can influence the calculation of conversion ratio as well. Ratios of 1:2.5 to 1:3 were mostly suggested (Kasir et al. 2013, Elridy et al. 2018, Lorenc et al. 2013, Dashtipour et al. 2016). The ratio of conversion between ABO and INCO has been more and more inclining to 1:2.5 recently.

CLINICAL OBSERVATION AMONG BOTULINUM TOXIN A PRODUCTS IN AESTHETIC PRACTICES

If there are two products of botulinum toxin A having equal clinical efficacy and potency, the active functioning molecules of botulinum toxin in the two different brand kits should be almost the same in amount after dissociation in physiological pH. But they can be different in terms of the total amount of toxin (some toxins are denatured), different in molecular weight (some are complexed with other protein units), and different in terms of the microenvironment (formulation, excipient, manufacturing method, and reconstitution). When the active units of botulinum toxin A from different brand kits have the same sequence of peptide chains and their binding to neural end plates and internalization to the nerve endings are not related with the complex and milieu that could be influenced by the toxin formulation, the difference of different kits could impact would be the spread and distribution of toxin molecules in tissue. When a hypothesis is true, that microscopic point of view should be compatible with clinical data. However, our assumption of being equal or not, simply based on the number of units and the grading scores given by the raters or patients, is still arbitrary. Toxin formulation and the excipients constitute the milieu can affect toxin character indeed, even with the same amount of active molecules in the same volume of toxin fluid. For example, the human serum albumin stabilizes toxin peptide and can have an impact on toxin performance in different laboratory conditions. Thought the conclusions from different studies on the spreading tendencies of different brand toxin kits are conflicting, the differences in spreading character and subjective feelings toward toxin effect are easily detectable. The temporary milieu of injected toxin in tissue determines the spreading tendency. Concentration, as most understand, is one of the factors. Toxin with less spreading tendency may work similarly in small muscles to one that is easily spreadable but might appear less effective in a broader muscle because of the reduced coverage when the points of injection are limited. That scenario does happen in daily practice and occurs more commonly in big muscles (see Chapter 16), as in injections for forehead wrinkles and the masseter (Figure 4.5). Stability of a toxin formulation might interfere with the equalness of its effect when compared with other products at different point of time after toxin reconstitution.

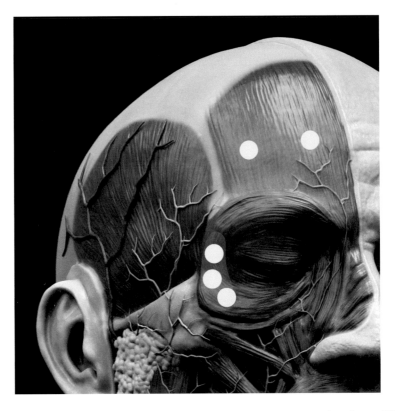

FIGURE 4.5   The toxin dose per injection spot and the reconstitution concentration do not differ too much for the forehead lines and for the crow's feet. The area of the crow's feet to be covered by the toxin is extremely small compared to the broad forehead area.

Spreading tendency could have impacts on the reading of clinical efficacy when the condition of a study involves more toxin distribution, for example, on the forehead.

BIBLIOGRAPHY

Ahn BK, et al. Consensus recommendations on the aesthetic usage of botulinum toxin type A in Asians. *Dermatol Surg* 2013;39:1843–1860.

Bradshaw M, et al. Regulation of neurotoxin complex expression in Clostridium botulinum strains 62A, Hall A-hyper, and NCTC 2916. *Anaerobe* 2004;10(6):321–333.

Bigalke H, Rummel A. Botulinum neurotoxins: Qualitative and quantitative analysis using the mouse phrenic nerve hemidiaphragm assay (MPN). *Toxins (Basel)* 2015 7(12):4895–4905.

Dashtipour K, Chen JJ, Espay AJ, Mari Z, Ondo W. OnabotulinumtoxinA and AbobotulinumtoxinA dose conversion: A systematic literature review. *Mov Disord Clin Pract.* 2016 3(2):109–115.

Dineen SS, et al. Neurotoxin gene clusters in Clostridium botulinum type A strains: sequence comparison and evolutionary implications. *Curr Microbiol* 2003;46(5):345–352.

Dressler D, et al. Measuring the potency labelling of OnabobotulinumtoxinA (Botox®) and IncobotulinumtoxinA (Xeomin®) in an LD50 assay. *J Neural Transm* 2012;119:13–15.

Elridy AS, et al. Comparison of the clinical efficacy of Abobotulinumtoxin A (Abobotulinumtoxin) and Onabobotulinumtoxin A (Ona) in the treatment of crow's feet wrinkles: A split-face study. *Semin Ophthalmol* 2018;33(6):739–747.

Fernández-Salas E, et al. Botulinum neurotoxin serotype A specific cell-based potency assay to replace the mouse bioassay. *PLoS One* 2012;7(11):e49516.

Field M, et al. AbobotulinumtoxinA (Dysport®), OnabobotulinumtoxinA (Botox®), and IncobotulinumtoxinA (Xeomin®) neurotoxin content and potential implications for duration of response in patients. *Toxins* 2018;10:535 pii: E535. doi: 10.3390/toxins10120535

First ER, et al. Dose standardisation of botulinum toxin. *Lancet* 1994;343:1035.

Frevert J. Content of botulinum neurotoxin in Botox(R)/Vistabel(R), Dysport(R)/Azzalure(R), and Xeomin(R)/Bocouture(R). *Drugs R D* 2010;10:67–73.

Frevert J. Pharmaceutical, biological, and clinical properties of Botulinum. *Drugs R D* 2015;15:1–9.

Frevert J, et al. Complexing proteins in botulinum toxin type A drugs: A help or a hindrance? *Biologics* 2010;4:325–332.

Frevert J, et al. Presence of clostridial DNA in botulinum toxin products. *Toxicon* 2015;93(suppl.):S28–S41.

Goodnough, et al. Stabilization of botulinum toxin type A during lyophilization. *Appl Environ Microbiol* 1992;58:3426–35.

Goschel H, et al. Botulinum A toxin therapy: Neutralizing and nonneutralizing antibodies – therapeutic consequences. *Exp Neurol* 1997;147(1):96–102.

Hambleton P, et al. Potency equivalence of botulinum toxin preparations. *J R Soc Med* 1994;87:719.

Hunt T, Clarke K. Potency evaluation of a formulated drug product containing 150-kd botulinum neurotoxin type A. *Clin Neuropharmacol* 2009;32(1):28–31.

Kane MAC, et al. A randomized, double-blind trial to investigate the equivalence of incobotulinumtoxinA and onabotulinumtoxinA for glabellar frown lines. *Dermatol Surg* 2015, 41(11):1310–1319.

Kassir R, et al. Triple-blind, prospective, internally controlled comparative study between AbobotulinumtoxinbotulinumtoxinA and OnabobotulinumtoxintulinumtoxinA for the treatment of Facial Rhytids. *Dermatol Ther (Heidelb)* 2013 Dec;3(2):179–189.

Kutschenko A, et al. The role of human serum albumin and neurotoxin associated proteins in the formulation of BoNT/A products. *Toxicon* 2019;168:158–163.

Lorenc ZP, et al. Consensus panel's assessment and recommendations on the use of 3 botulinum toxin type A products in facial aesthetics. *Aesthet Surg J* 2013;33 (1 Suppl):35S-40S.

Michael A, et al. A randomized, double-blind trial to investigate the equivalence of IncobotulinumtoxinA and OnabobotulinumtoxinA for glabellar frown lines. *Dermatol Surg* 2015;41(11):1310–1319.

Moers-Carpi M, et al. A randomised, double-blind comparison of 20 units of onabotulinumtoxinA with 30 units of incobotulinumtoxinA for glabellar lines. *J Cosmet Laser Ther* 2012;14(6):296–303.

Muti G, Harrington L. A prospective rater and subject blinded study comparing the efficacy of incobotulinumtoxinA and onabotulinumtoxintulinumtoxinA to treat crow's feet: A clinical crossover evaluation. *Dermatol Surg.* 2015 Jan;41(Suppl 1):S39–S46.

Pan L, et al. Comparing lanbotulinumtoxinA (Hengli®) with OnabobotulinumtoxinA (Botox®) and IncobotulinumtoxinA (Xeomin®) in the mouse hemidiaphragm assay. *J Neural Transm (Vienna)* 2019;126(12):1625–1629.

Panjwani N, et al. Biochemical, functional and potency characteristics of type A botulinum toxin in clinical use. *Botulinum J* 2008;1(1):153–166.

Prager W, et al. Botulinum toxin type A treatment to the upper face: Retrospective analysis of daily practice. *Clin Cosmet Investig Dermatol* 2012;5:53–8.

Prager W, et al. Incobotulinumtoxin a for aesthetic indications: A systematic review of prospective comparative trials. *Dermatol Surg* 2017;(7):959–966.

Sattler G, et al. Noninferiority of IncobotulinumtoxinA, free from complexing proteins, compared with another botulinum toxin type A in the treatment of glabellar frown lines. *Dermatol Surg* 2010;36(Suppl 4):2146–2154.

Schantz EJ, Johnson EA. Properties and use of botulinum toxin and other microbial neurotoxins in medicine. *Microbiol Rev* 1992;56:80–99.

Schellekens H, Casadevall N. Immunogenicity of recombinant human proteins: Causes and consequences. *J Neurol* 2004;251(Suppl 2):114–119.

Van den Bergh P, et al. (1996) Dose standardisation of BTX. In: 3rd International Dystonia Symposium, 9–11 October, 1996, Miami, Florida. Affiliated National Dystonia Associations, Chicago, p 30.

Whitemarsh RC, et al. Novel application of human neurons derived from induced pluripotent stem cells for highly sensitive botulinum neurotoxin detection. *Toxicol Sci* 2012;126:426–435.

Zbinden G, et al. Significance of the LD50-test for the toxicological evaluation of chemical substances. *Arch Toxicol.* 1981;47(2):77–99.

5 The Aesthetic Standard for Contouring and Facial Dynamics

Yates Yen-Yu Chao

CONTENTS

The development of modern aesthetic medicine owes much to the tiny molecule of botulinum toxin, which works among the numerous nerve endings extending to the muscle fibers and skin appendages. Its modern uses can be traced back to the incidental finding when it was used in the treatment of blepharospasm. Glabellar frowning wrinkles decreased along with the modulation of external ocular muscles. The rapid and noticeable effacement of deeply carved wrinkles days after the administration of a tiny amount of a pharma liquid was just like a miracle initiated under the sway of a magic wand that stopped or enhanced some normal movements focally.

With the commercialization of procedures, people have been persuaded by and believe in their effects in terms of rejuvenation and the improvement of outward appearance. That motivates their investment in purchasing injections and using toxin doses for the enhancement of beauty. However, the magic can work in an opposite direction. It has yet to be determined if the immobilization of facial units equates to attractiveness or youthfulness.

WHAT ARE WRINKLES BLAMED FOR?

Wrinkles appear from the initial dynamic contraction of mimetic muscles that pull or squeeze facial soft tissues as dynamic lines. After years of folding, these temporary lines turned into permanent

DOI: 10.1201/9781003008132-5

indented marks. The deep dents that persist symbolize age and show the traces of repeated muscle action. However, wrinkles, especially the dynamic ones, suggest also the normal dynamicity of the face and, of course, the expressions, moods, emotions, and well-being of the subject. Dynamic movements and expressive folds are inherent and normal since birth; contour lines around the eyes and the modiolus of the mouth are natural and would not be interpreted as signifying age when they appear in adolescents. When treating wrinkles, we have to realize there is nothing wrong with the movements of mimetic muscles or the folds and lines that relate to muscle contraction. It is not the line itself but the pattern of these lines and the presentation of the neighboring structures that suggest tissue laxity and soft-tissue sagginess.

THE ROLE OF TOXIN IN WRINKLE REDUCTION

The muscles that we tackle with toxins in order to reduce wrinkles are the same ones governing our expressions, transmitting signals and messages to the world. When analyzing these lines on a smiling youthful face and those on an old face, it can be quickly found that the differences between them are not that they exist in one and not the other, or even that they differ in their depth or extent, but in the pattern implying or appearing as a part of the aging process (Figure 5.1a,b). The pattern of wrinkles that transmit a message of aging includes the amount, density, array, depth, curving, distribution, and neighboring tissue bulging and/or sagging, distortion and/or traction, depression, and rippling. That means that the annihilation of muscle movements alone does not transform an old-looking face into a youthful one. However, the eradication of focal facial movements or the immobilization of selective facial landmarks makes a face look strange (Figure 5.2a,b,c). The correction of an aged pattern with toxin should be directed toward the moderation of movement rather than toward stopping movement.

In treatment, the range or magnitude of muscle excursion should be modified wisely and artistically to match the agreed ideal age and the whole facial presentation. The other treatment modalities should be designed and employed as part of a whole package – a comprehensive treatment plan that solves the problems rather than just inhibiting the muscle function only.

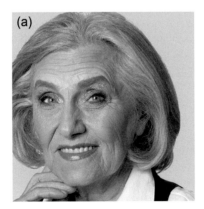
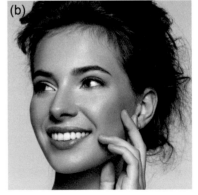

FIGURE 5.1 Nasolabial folds present in both aged (a) and young women (b). They are often regarded as a sign of aging and patients ask for them to be removed through treatments. However, they are a normal facial contour and suggest smiles and positive expressions. It is the neighboring tissue curves, the nearby skin quality, the fullness of the cheeks, and the folding pattern that determine whether a nasolabial fold appears to be sign of aging or not.

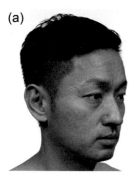 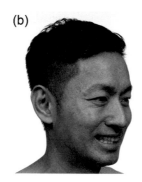 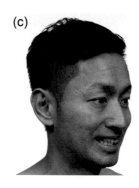

FIGURE 5.2   Facial expressions are composite movements of multiple facial structures. Using graphic software, the upper face of (a) is merged with the smiling lower face (b), forming into the odd image of (c), which resembles the toxin faces we encounter that combine a partial smile with an incompatibly serene periorbital zone.

NEGATIVE EXPRESSIONS AND NEGATIVE MUSCLES?

Pharmaceutical muscle modulation is an innovation claimed to modify expressions and mood. The original ambition of control over the consequence of muscle contraction has further evolved into controlling the muscle function and, more specifically, the expressing function. The muscle functions to be deleted are the expressions classified as negative. Arguably, aesthetic judgment or intervention is in danger of having gone too far in trying to define which expressions should be called negative. Is the removal of part of a normal facial contour or part of normal expressive ability not like some mutilating surgeries that cut nerves or muscles to fit ideals corresponding to a certain period of life or morphological pattern? Destructive procedures that sacrifice the normal function of normal structures like walking or core muscle balance would be regarded as an ethical issue. In a similar way, the annihilation of a patient's outlets to express anger or grief seems inhuman. If it is the same muscular system in our face that governs both movements delivering messages and the pressure forming wrinkles, we should adjust our goals and doses carefully to level down the strength and extent of muscle excursion instead of to prevent it totally.

PARALYZED BEAUTY AND DISTORTED ELEGANCY

As botulinum toxin became more and more popular, it became routine for aesthetic medical enhancement and its use has evolved into more and more diversified clinical usage. Unfortunately, it also became easy to spot which faces might have had toxin treatment recently or too much or badly. Let's look back to the initial intention we gave and the patient's request for the toxin. Did they really want to tell others that toxin has been applied to their faces? And do they really think those faces where the use of toxin is recognizable are more beautiful (see Figure 5.2c)? How can even laypersons tell that something has been done and know it was not good enough (see Chapter 6)?

Most patients who request or undergo routine toxin treatment had completely normal facial movements originally. However, the additional modification or erasure of facial muscle function could turn normal into abnormal. We all learn visual communication from birth and know well what a normal facial movement pattern is. That is how we read nonverbal messages and know when things have happened to our friends such as facial palsy and of course, actual iatrogenic, unexplained facial immobility, or the incoherence of facial subunits.

The treatment to completely paralyze a muscle unit is not difficult. A strategic titration and distribution of toxin, considering the whole facial balance and expressive functions, is much more an art that adjusts the muscular activities out of normal but within the normal range, releasing the muscles that have been hypertonic or hyperkinetic, balancing the imbalanced muscle groups by suppressing the overactive and overprominent ones, modifying the pattern of synergy for more elegance, reducing the amplitude of an area while keeping the original harmony, and masking some suboptimals like asymmetry, traumatic sequelae, and contour/functional restrictions. The injection of toxin could then be considered a treatment that walks the line between disease and appearance and modestly diminishes and disguises the signs of aging.

DYNAMIC WRINKLES AND EXPRESSIONS

The art of wrinkle management is not to remove but to modify, reduce, and improve them; the philosophy of toxin treatment is to reduce and modify muscle activity while keeping their functional balance and expressiveness.

BROW POSITION AND SHAPE

Brow position and shape are innately related to patterned brow hair distribution and to brow bone and fat prominence. The brow is dynamically raised, dragged down, or lessened by surrounding muscles. Aging is a process that involves possible ligament loosening, bone resorption, and fat/soft-tissue sagging. The toxin that raises the downward displacement or changes the original shape of the eyebrow actually modifies the opposing balance among muscles or creates a new balance. Symmetric dosing is extremely important. Dosing should be modest in view of muscle synergism.

EYE APERTURE

The toxin has been used for the orbicularis oculi fibers close to the lower eyelid margin, mildly releasing the closure and changing the lower lid curve pattern and the degree of eye-opening. Dosing here should be extremely minimal at the point showing overcontraction or the point of a reverse eyelid upturn. Treatment should be reserved only for cases with excessive muscle contraction that distorts the smooth eyelid curve or excessive upward shielding of the eyeball during a smile.

MASSETER

Masseter toxin injection should be restricted to the lower portion, preserving normal masticating function. Further refining the technique of masseter treatment should involve adaptive designs tailoring the injection points in accordance with the morphological requirements (see Chapter 18).

MOUTH CORNER

Toxin blocking the downward-pulling muscles could in compensation enhance the elevators that pull the mouth corner up. Conservative dosing should be emphasized for those showing hypertonic depressor activities. Interventions that disrupt the normal balance around the mouth modiolus would possibly result in a strange stationary and dynamic mouth shape and could potentially interfere with normal pronunciation.

BODY: CALF

Toxin to treat the calf is usually needed in greater doses than for labeled aesthetic use because the gastrocnemius and soleus muscles are much bigger in size. The function of the target muscles is crucial for body movement and posture support. The suppression of normal calf function along with the requirement of high toxin doses increase its controversial aspects. Treatment should be conservative in dosing and properly aimed for contouring rather than affecting the activity of the entire muscle. Injections should be limited to bulging parts only to maintain intact the normal functions of standing, walking, and running.

BODY: BACK AND SHOULDER

There are similar concerns here as for the calf muscles. The requirement of mobility function and central axial body balance are all essentials for these trunk muscles, outweighing any other pursuits of a better shape.

FOREHEAD

The frontalis muscle contracts to pull up the structures that are connected with the insertion fibers. Forehead contraction raises and moves the brow, eyelids, and the neighboring soft tissue like a curtain. The attachment of muscle fiber concentrates more at the end of the brow, which dimples the skin where the ligamentous structure attaches to the orbital rim. The raising force shows different strengths and vectors from medial to lateral and varies between individuals. Squeezing of the soft tissue and skin in the span of the frontalis forces them into skin folds and grooves. The above variables, along with the condition of the skin and soft tissue, make the winding grooves deeper and more curving in areas being squeezed more. This wrinkling pattern reflects well the dynamics of individual muscle exercising, and that is an important part of personal features. This wrinkling pattern is closely associated with the movement of brows that draws visual attention like flags.

   Toxin treatment for the forehead is a common practice. Knowing the distribution of the frontalis muscle that lays on the frontal bone is not difficult and can be carried out through visual observation of the distribution of dynamic wrinkles and through hand palpation. To eliminate them totally by thorough toxin administration and chasing for residual wrinkles would be straightforward and can be easily imagined if the information about the extent of toxin spread for muscles can be identified. But to have frozen facial structures is not ideal and should not be the goal of forehead toxin treatment. Instead, treatment at the next level should respect the original pattern of muscle distribution and movement and be better at maintaining facial expressions, keeping the original brow alignment without overcompromising the compensatory raising of the eyebrow in patients with sagging, tissue redundancy, or eyebrow/eyelid ptosis (see Chapter 14).

FROWN

Frowning is the movement where multiple muscles contract within or near the glabella complex. Usually, the vector contributed by the main role of the corrugator is toward the center and mildly inferiorly. However, in practice, different patterns of synergism exist among the nearby muscles including fibers of the frontalis, orbicularis oculi, procerus, depressor supercilii, nasalis, and the multiple mouth levators. Approximation of the brow is an important part of various expressions, including frowning. These related muscles govern the movements of the surrounding structures and especially the brows. The imbalance among the multiple complex opponents occurs when one of these members is inhibited by the toxin. In addition to pulling upward and downward, tension is maintained between the medial and the lateral components. Compensatory hyperfunction happens when one of the opponents becomes weaker (Figure 5.3). The position and shape of related structures are other issues of concern when having toxin treatment in this area.

   Some long-term dynamic wrinkles would turn permanent and visible without muscle contraction. These permanent prints of muscle activity should be also filled with fillers to seal the gaps (see Chapter 17).

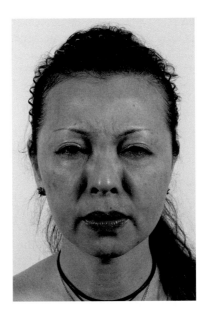

FIGURE 5.3 Frowning movements often involve the glabella complex muscles and the neighboring muscles, including frontalis, nasalis, orbicularis oculi, etc. After toxin blocking of the corrugator and procerus, minimal residual contraction of these two muscles is visible while the contraction of medial orbicularis oculi and levator labii muscles is apparent as well. Expressions from these rearranged muscle movements are puzzling and quite unlike any of the patterns we are familiar with.

Crow's Feet

Crow's feet are the lines under muscle contraction over the lateral corner of the eye. The target muscle of toxin injection is the lateral part of the orbicularis oculi muscle that surrounds the eye aperture to effect eye closure. These dynamic wrinkles, conveying messages of smiling and laughter, are not bad features to be eliminated. However, aging can intensify these lines in depth and extent and change their pattern as a sign of aging. Traditionally, it is recommended that the orbicularis oculi is injected near the brim of the bony orbit, but these lines extend far more over the infraorbital region, across the zygomatic arch, and lateral to the temple.

Positive messages of joyfulness and happiness should not be deleted with these injections. A dynamic circle that has become broken with part of it paralyzed after toxin treatment looks somehow diseased. Compensation could occur that further ruins the picture and magnifies the contrast. Chasing the lines with toxin must be done carefully as some of the medial extension of toxin injection could interfere with the eyelid closing function and worsen the problem of an eyelid bag. Lower placement of toxin across the zygoma could work on mouth elevators. For patients with broad orbicularis oculi, however, the standard protocols of injection appear short in coverage.

An artistic approach to introducing toxin to the lateral orbital lines should be personalized according to wrinkle pattern and distribution. Carefully maintaining muscle activities could retain the expression of excitement while improving elegance.

Lifting

Botulinum toxin has been used for facial lifting for a couple of years. The mechanism behind toxin lifting is to block the depressor muscles that pull the tissue down, reserving the opponents of the elevator to pull the tissues and facial landmarks up. It is easy to see that movements of facial structures play between the opposing muscles. When the balance between opponents is favored toward one side, the movement pattern can also be changed. Some of the landmark position or orientation changes become odd in appearance after muscle lifting. That kind of elevation could not even be considered as enhancement or improvement. The other concern is the short duration of botulinum toxin and its reproducibility if the elevation comes from temporary muscle inhibition. Practitioners should judge its feasibility based on these factors (see Chapter 14).

BIBLIOGRAPHY

Beebe B, et al. A systems view of mother–infant face-to-face communication. *Dev Psychol* 2016;52(4):556–571.

Braadbaart L, et al. The shared neural basis of empathy and facial imitation accuracy. *Neuroimage* 2014;84:367–375.

Cattaneo L, et al. The facial motor system. *Neurosci Biobehav Rev* 2014;38:135–159.

Hsu CT, et al. Enhanced emotional and motor responses to live versus videotaped dynamic facial expressions. *Sci Rep* 2020;10(1):16825.

Ishai A, et al. Face perception is mediated by a distributed cortical network. *Brain Res Bull* 2005;67(1–2):87–93.

Lackey JN, et al. Implications of botulinum toxin injection of the brow. *J Am Acad Dermatol* 2006;54(5):921–922.

Lewis MB. Exploring the positive and negative implications of facial feedback. *Emotion* 2012;12(4):852–859.

Lewis MB. The interactions between botulinum-toxin-based facial treatments and embodied emotions. *Sci Rep* 2018;8(1):14720.

Michaud T, et al. Facial dynamics and emotional expressions in facial aging treatments. *J Cosmet Dermatol* 2015;14(1):9–21.

Neal DT, et al. Embodied emotion perception: Amplifying and dampening facial feedback modulates emotion perception accuracy. *Soc Psychol Pers Sci* 2011;2(6):673–678.

6 To Immobilize or Modulate Muscle Function?

Yates Yen-Yu Chao

CONTENTS

When the result of an aesthetic botulinum toxin treatment can be easily recognized as such, there must be something we can detect that deviates from normal. Interestingly, these traits of abnormality can be easily detected by laypeople without professional knowledge of facial muscle structures and dynamics. For a subject's friends and acquaintances who detect the differences, the awareness can be attributed to the comparison of the original muscle exercising pattern they are used to and the new one that presents after the toxin treatment. But with the examples we encounter for the first time on screen or in real life, we still can tell. There must be something conflicting with the rules we learned since birth – the pattern of normal human facial movements. Facial muscle synergism works in various patterns, as documented in the literature, but most of us can compile these patterns as normal. How could this various weirdness trigger an alarm in our systems of recognition? There must be something outside the usual database of visual communication. When similar messages are sent to medical practitioners who have a better understanding of the underlying neuromuscular function and mechanism, they should diagnose any error or signs of manipulation much more easily and quickly than the public, as they are aware of the usual rules as well.

In this chapter, the usual suboptimal results in aesthetic toxin practice are outlined and described, including their underlying reasons and the key steps to avoiding these errors.

FROZEN FACE

Botulinum toxin treatment for aesthetic purposes should be anything but intended to immobilize the face. Muscle functions for expression and communication are essential and should not be blocked totally. Frozen faces can be debilitated focally, regionally, asymmetrically, or uniformly; they are not acceptable and should be avoided.

The goal of wrinkle treatment should be to ameliorate the magnitude or strength of muscle contraction, instead of completely eradicating it. A high dose or large unit per shot quietens the muscle fibers within the spreading diameter. Multiple shots of a large unit in a specific region often complete denervate that area temporarily. The goal of contour correction is different. Masseter blocking should be as complete as possible but only on part of the muscle (lower third). The doses for brow or mouth corner elevation should be minimal, allowing for further fine adjustment or boosting.

DOI: 10.1201/9781003008132-6

NONCOHERENT DYNAMICITY

When the degree of muscle movement decreases after toxin inhibition, muscles remain functional but less active. In those circumstances, a set of muscle movements that is composed of several components could become noncoherent and discernible; one area might show exercise much less than the others, and this discrepancy can be detectable.

The discrepancy usually consists of some muscle groups with normal activity and other muscles with damped action. The discrepancy, with its focal suppressed response to reasonable emotional reaction, is another reason why the face can seem strange. When synergism (see The section "Neglect of Synergy" below) (Figures 6.1, 6.2) involves the muscle that has been treated, compensatory hyperactivity usually further highlights this discrepancy.

The aim of an aesthetic treatment with toxin injection would be to administer doses moderately and respect the pattern of muscle synergism. Physical examination should include visual observation of muscle excursion and palpable evaluation of muscle strength. The synergistic muscle should be treated in addition to the actual target muscles.

UNBALANCED TENSION

Mimetic muscles contract and pull facial structures in a vector compliant to their orientation. A facial structure with multiple muscle insertions behaves like a pivot, with multiple forces pulling in different directions. These complex mechanical forces are kept in a dynamic and tensional balance. Similar models apply to this principle and could work in a more complicated pattern with muscle attachment at different parts of a structure.

This balance could be changed by weakening one of these vectors. Consequences after the break of balance include tissue dislocation, distortion, deviation, compensatory overaction, and crooked movements.

Injection of the toxin is targeted at certain problems, and the injection often follows the rule on several typical points. Spock's eyebrow is one of the examples (Figure 6.3). Differential dosing for the frontalis muscle results in an imbalance between medial and lateral fibers. The eyebrow tilts under the imbalance, and the lateral end of the eyebrow is elevated. Balance has to be kept not only

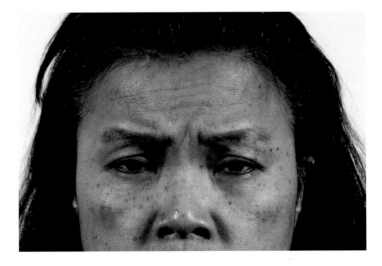

FIGURE 6.1 The synergism of frontalis and corrugator occurs when this patient frowns, resulting in concomitant glabella and forehead lines.

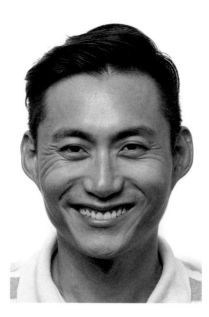

FIGURE 6.2 Smile movements often involve the muscle of orbicularis oculi and levator muscles including zygomaticus major and minor, risorius, nasalis and dilator naris, etc.

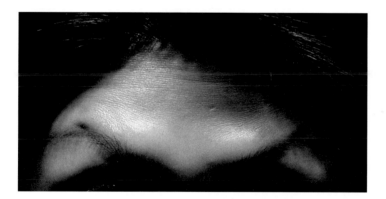

FIGURE 6.3 Spock's deformity occurs when unpaired muscle activities are produced through toxin treatment.

across the frontalis but also between the elevator and the depressors. Imbalance can occur when the opponents of this antagonism are being treated in preference to one side (Figure 6.4).

Muscles of the glabella complex pull the eyebrow in different directions. Toxin dosing among these muscles should be balanced as well to keep the brow in its original orientation and retain the normal movement direction. Medial depressor muscles counteract both the medial elevating frontalis fibers and the lateral pulling forces. That is why when glabella muscle inhibition is complete, the pivotal structure of the eyebrow moves slightly laterally and upward. The intereyebrow distance can become wider; the arch of the eyebrow can be emphasized and become prominent.

Toxin treatments for structures with multivector opponents need to be calculated with regard to the relative loss and gain and administered with preventive measures to avoid the mismatch. Minimal doses of toxin should be applied to the point where compensatory hyperfunction could be anticipated. These patients should be closely followed up after the procedure and the treatment

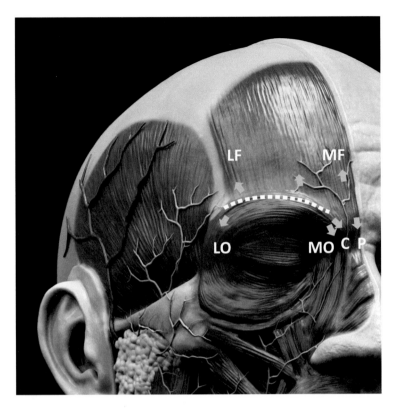

FIGURE 6.4 There are several mechanisms that can occur during the treatment of botulinum toxin resulting in Spock's brow deformity. They are the imbalance between the medial and lateral muscle activity; either the medial or lateral activity is the net vector among the multiple forces.

area can be touched up if any imbalance has occurred. Any touch-up injection should be conservative to avoid another reverse imbalance. Usually, this reverse imbalance is not easy to correct. For new patients who have never received this treatment before, practitioners could evaluate the relative muscle strength by hand palpation and muscle countercontraction. Dosing based on experience is important, and it is best to be conservative. For patients whom you have treated previously, detailed documentation of the injection points and doses will help you modify the treatment plan at the next treatment. Responses of these muscles after the treatment are valuable information for further adjustment. Patients who have been treated elsewhere previously should be carefully asked about their experiences and preferences, and this should be followed up with an objective comparison.

NEGLECT OF SYNERGY

Synergism is a common phenomenon where a group of muscles is innervated in a parallel connection. The parallel innervation could be strongly associated or partially connected. When a signal from the nervous system arrives, these muscles work together as a group. Synergism plays an important role in completing a movement such as swallowing or sneezing and in different facial expressions. Closer observation of these synergies of facial mimetic muscles ca reveal minor differences among individuals. When one component of the group is suppressed, the other members in the same group keep on responding to the command, and the presented movements change in pattern.

Toxin treatment without taking muscle synergy into account could lead to isolated or compensatory muscle contraction. These contractions usually become prominent against a relatively quiet toxin-touched background. For example, facial frowning in some patients involves frontalis fibers.

Compensatory action of the frontalis could result in paradoxical contraction of the forehead in patients who have been treated for the frown without concomitant attention to the forehead.

Close observation is the key to a successful treatment involving synergistic myogroups. Usually, a treatment using botulinum toxin has muscle as the key target, and appropriate doses of the toxin should be placed on the key muscle. When synergism is strong, the other contributing muscles should be considered for modulation as well. These contributing muscles can be classified as adjuvant muscles, which function in a similar way and in a similar direction; corresponding muscles, which function in a different way but contribute together as a complete performance; and opponent muscles, which counteract with the muscle and often provide tension to achieve a dynamic balance. An artistic treatment should respect the importance of each role played in the synergism and allocate gradient doses to achieve a new harmonic balance.

IRRATIONAL CONTOURS

Many of our facial contours are maintained by background structural muscle tone. The normal muscular function provides the mechanical basis for projection, curves, and dimension. However, toxin treatment can interfere with these functions and weaken these mechanics, resulting in strange contours. For example, toxin injection has been used to increase mouth pout or the opening of the orbital aperture. However, dosing only slightly beyond the minimal range could result in flappy lips or scleral show. Droopy curves, incompetent close, dysfunction, and movement lag could accompany the fault as well.

Off-label use of toxin should be explored extremely cautiously because any suboptimal results could be more open to blame and liability. Some toxin treatments adjusting static facial contours are potentially close to being dangerous, as many delicate structures and functions are intricately maintained by physiological neuromuscular networks.

Practitioners must be aware that the toxin effect lasts only for some months and gradually loses its effect over this period of time. It does not seem sensible to attempt static contour adjustment of a fundamentally mobile mechanism throughout the initial dynamic block and recovery period.

INCOMPLETE OR UNEVEN DOSING

When a toxin treatment has been done following the advice to maintain reasonable muscle function and interrelated harmonious balance, the minimal amount of toxin can still be applied unevenly. A homogeneous toxin effect should be the combination of enough points of injection together with appropriate dosage and point-to-point separations. A broad muscle span or a big block of bulky muscle all need to be evenly treated with adequate and even toxin coverage. The number of units per shot vary according to the character of a specific toxin, and the volume of reconstitution is related to the extent of toxin spread.

Sometimes an incomplete toxin effect happens because the toxin cannot reach the target of the motor end plate efficiently. The administration of the toxin is often not done directly to the target itself or is not close enough. When we carefully examine what is considered as common practice, the toxin is often delivered through tissue diffusion, with limited points of injection, in large units but through few injection points, through intradermal injection aiming for intramuscular action, etc. Thick muscles, like masseter, with compartments, can be blocked incompletely if the injection is not delivered at different depths and to different compartments. Freestyle injections of toxin can interrupt muscle contraction unevenly when the shots of toxin are administered randomly in spatial arrangement, in injection depth, or in dose, and this type of treatment would need to rely greatly on touch-up corrections.

The depth of injection, number of points, dosing, and spatial arrangement require a precise calculation, not a repeat of a standard protocol or merely the work of injection. Where and how much toxin is used matters.

ASYMMETRY

Asymmetry happens quite often and occurs more than most expect. However, these minor faults are often more prominent shortly after the onset of the toxin effects. It seems that many toxin patients are not called back for check-up. Even though the injection of the toxin on a symmetrical face should be just a mirror repeat of the first side, various factors can supervene and be the reason for asymmetry (Figure 6.5). This error will be elaborated on further in Chapter 8.

OVERDOSING OR FALSE TARGETING

A precise botulinum toxin treatment should be appropriate in terms of dosing and delivered exactly to the movement center without interfering with the neighboring tissue and irrelevant muscle activities. However, errors can happen when the peptides flood across into innocent muscle fibers or the parcel of pharma protein is delivered to the wrong address. That happens more often when the amount of injected toxin is more than is necessary, overdiluted, or overspread; or if the needle is inserted at a point not appropriate in depth or location, and the bevel used is not the best in direction and angle.

Many traditional injection techniques using high doses per shot in limited injection points work through toxin spread. Spread might help cover a bigger target muscle but cannot avoid also having an impact on the muscles close by. This phenomenon frequently happens in areas where muscle structures are complex, stratified, and sit closely together. The glabella and medial orbit have the muscles for frowning, for eye closure, for eyelid elevation, and for eyeball movements. Lateral orbit orbicularis oculi fibers are also close to the muscles of the zygomaticus muscle group, which elevate the cheek soft tissue. Injections for the perioral depressors and the superficial or medial shots for the masseter could all reach muscles nearby, resulting in unwanted effects.

To lessen the extent of toxin spread, the toxin could be reconstituted with less saline, composing a thicker solution. The same dosage could be split into more dabs with fewer units. The injection must be tailored according to the target muscle depth and be as close as possible to the muscle itself. The injection must be done extremely carefully in areas where muscles overlap in structure.

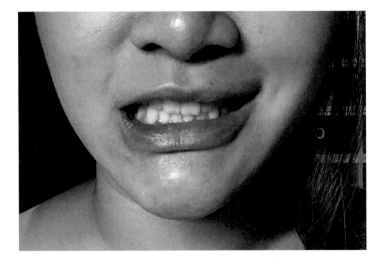

FIGURE 6.5 The depth and location of toxin injections are important for lower face treatments because the perioral muscles are stratified in layers without prominent surface landmarks. Minor deviations may result in incorrect targeting and unwanted asymmetric results.

BIBLIOGRAPHY

Ferreira MC, et al. Complications with the use of botulinum toxin type A in facial rejuvenation: Report of 8 cases. *Aesthetic Plast Surg* 2004;28(6):441–444.

Flynn TC. Advances in the use of botulinum neurotoxins in facial esthetics. *J Cosmet Dermatol* 2012;11(1):42–50.

Foissac R, et al. Influence of botulinum toxin type A esthetic injections on facial expressions. *J Cosmet Dermatol* 2021;20(5):1405–1410.

Iozzo I, et al. Multipoint and multilevel injection technique of botulinum toxin A in facial aesthetics. *J Cosmet Dermatol* 2014;13(2):135–142.

Sommer B. How to avoid complications when treating hyperdynamic folds and wrinkles. *Clin Dermatol* 2003;21(6):521–523.

Vartanian AJ, et al. Complications of botulinum toxin A use in facial rejuvenation. *Facial Plast Surg Clin North Am* 2005;13(1):1–10.

7 Achieving Better Results through Proper Instrumentation for Aesthetic Toxin Practice

Yates Yen-Yu Chao

CONTENTS

Compared with other inject-form drugs and injectable fillers, botulinum toxin injections are relatively small in scale and need more fastidious precision. Similar to injectable fillers, the depth of injection is closely related to the final therapeutic and aesthetic effects and has to be scrupulously controlled. But the effect of the injectable toxin is very different from that of injectable fillers, in that it has its onset several days later, with an exponential magnification of functions rather than a real-time measurable and detectable inflation of volume. After the effects have happened, it is not easy to reverse or erase them quickly. That is why every deployment of toxin must be judicious, while the precise delivery of the pharma protein has to be accomplished with the appropriate injecting instruments.

SYRINGE

In practice, insulin syringes and smaller volume syringes are mostly used for the injection of botulinum toxin, except for work for indications off the face. The manner of preparation, type of syringe, and size of syringe could all impact on the precision of toxin practice.

SIZE OF SYRINGE

The syringes most employed for toxin injection are 1 mL, 0.5 mL, and 0.3 mL-sized syringes (Figure 7.1). When the injection scale is about 1 unit of Ona or Inco, it becomes critical to control the injection in exactly the required amount (Figure 7.2). A one-grid push is usually the minimum volume practitioners could rely on for the control of aliquot size. According to the standard reconstitution

DOI: 10.1201/9781003008132-7

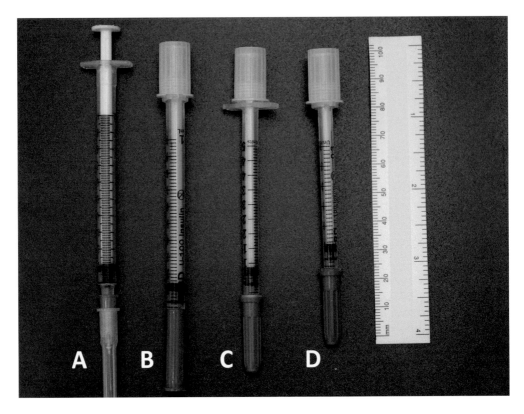

FIGURE 7.1 Syringes of smaller volume reduce the diameter of syringe and extend the fluid containing space, allowing for finer grids.

protocol for Onabotulinum toxin A, a total of 2.5 mL saline is added per bottle of 100-unit kit. So a full syringe of 1 mL standard reconstituted Onabotulinum toxin A contains 40 units of active toxin. Syringes with 5 grids are marked as 0.1 mL; one large grid (0.1 mL) equals 4 units, and one small grid (0.02 mL) is 0.8 units. Some of the 1 mL syringes have their graduations as fine as 0.01 mL but these are very tightly printed; discrimination and control with these very fine grids becomes difficult and impractical. Practitioners might not be able to stop precisely at the intended grid mark so that the expected precision turns out to be unattainable. As one grid represents 0.8 instead of 1 unit, I would not suggest the practitioner fit into the usual guidance based on integers by adding subjectively a little more than one grid. The subjective part beyond the grids can be too arbitrary, but the little difference, or imprecision, will become a reality. A better solution is to modify the recommendation of 2.5 mL to 2 mL and have the final solution be a little thicker. Then one grid represents 1 unit. Or just follow the usual teachings that are based on the unit by the grid. That means injecting 80% of what you learned while keeping all the allocations and proportions the same.

Beginners in administering botulinum toxin usually have to follow the guide first to know where to give toxin and the relative weight of dosage. It is not easy for them to adapt what they have learned into their personal techniques to disperse toxin in more points with fewer units.

Using syringes of smaller caliber could be beneficial for easier control in dispensing minimal doses of toxin. For standard 0.5 mL syringes, the fine grids of the syringe are further refined to represent 0.01 mL, i.e. 0.5 units of toxin when reconstituted with 2 mL of saline. The practitioner can better control the push of the plunger by one or two grids, delivering a smaller amount of toxin. Though imprecision could occur when stopping the plunger just right on the grid, any error could be less. That helps a lot when the same minimal doses are to be given symmetrically for bilateral

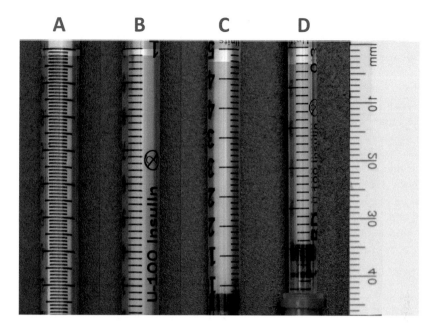

FIGURE 7.2   For the 1 mL insulin syringe with detachable needle (A), one small grid represents 0.01 mL. However, the grids are too close to be precisely controlled by plunger pushing. (B) The 1 mL insulin syringes with fixed short needles are equipped with similar grids but usually feature 5 grids per 0.1 mL. That means one grid represents 0.02 mL. The 0.5 mL (C) and 0.3 mL (D) insulin syringes are outfitted with fixed short needles and are labeled with 10 grids per 0.1 mL, with wider grids for the syringes containing smaller volume. This favors minimal dosing with better precision.

identical structures. Insulin syringes of 0.3 mL further narrow the instrument caliber and lengthen the distance between grids for fine dosing. For delicate and superficial structures, precision is much more attainable with these kits.

Type of Syringe

The syringes commonly used for botulinum toxin injection can be further classified into four types:

 i. PP (polypropylene)/PE (polyethylene) hypodermal syringe with fixed needle, 29, 30, or 31G;
 ii. PP/PE hypodermal syringe with Luer slip tip;
 iii. PP/PE hypodermal syringes with Luer lock tip;
 iv. PC (polycarbonate) hypodermal syringes with Luer lock tip.

The choice of syringes from different manufacturers is too plentiful to be covered, but they can be roughly categorized into these four types.

Syringes with a fixed needle extract the toxin drug by piercing through the stopper with the same needle that is then to be used for injection; that practice wears the needle, and a blunt needle hurts the patient more. The benefit of using syringes with a fixed needle is its tight closure system, which allows easier and better control over the plunger. There is less dead space after the whole expelling process. The problem of needle-wearing can be lessened by open bottle extraction without penetration through the stopper. The extraction procedure has to be careful to avoid contamination of the toxin solution, and the whole product has to be harvested in one step and as quickly as possible. Some practitioners prepare the injecting syringes together and store them in the fridge for further use. Toxin potency was observed to be similar after thawing to toxin that was never frozen. However, this preparation is not completely sterile, and the amount of toxin becomes fixed, not adaptable to the patients' requirements.

The problem with slip-tip syringes is the loose connection between the detachable needle and the syringe. If air is present anterior to the plunger within the syringe, the compressible air between the fluid adds imprecision to the injection process and will severely hamper the brake of the manual drive.

Resistance inside the syringe between the lumen and plunger is important to help the control of injection pushing movements. When the interface between the two is sleek, the plunger tends to speed too much on every advance and it becomes harder to brake. Grid-wise advancement becomes difficult and more injection errors happen. Generally speaking, the resistance is higher in syringes with a fixed needle and lowest in PC syringes. Even with tight fixing of the needle through a Luer lock, the plunger of the PC kit could easily slip over upon a soft push.

FILLING OF SYRINGES

For syringes with fixed needles, the toxin can be extracted with the stopper removed as described above. For syringes with detachable needles, toxin fluid could be extracted using a larger caliber needle and then injected with a fine needle. The needle should be tightly fixed to avoid leaks. Any air present inside the syringes should be completely expelled to ensure the drug is in a vacuumed air-free system. For a syringe with a Luer lock connector, the needle has to be tightly screwed up with any air expelled in a similar pattern as the slip tip one. The plunger should be controlled more slowly and cautiously.

NEEDLE

Needles are the invasive elements that actually get into tissues and deliver drugs. The caliber of the needle and sharpness of the tip are directly related to the pain of needle insertion, while the size of the needle hole and pattern of bevel have an impact on the amount and direction of drug outflow. The desired depth of injection is generally reachable even with the fixed needle of insulin syringes. However, for indications away from the face and large muscles, detachable needles with longer dimensions are preferable to finish the delivery.

SIZE OF NEEDLE

It is generally believed the size of the needle relates directly to the pain of injection. In fact, the pain of toxin injection can be classified into two parts.

Needle Pricking Pain

The minimal trauma on the skin surface sensitizes the skin nerve endings and results in pain. Usually, the disruption occurs on a smaller scale for finer needles, and the resulting pain is perceived as milder. Botulinum toxin is generally delivered by fine needles in the gauge of 29G or more. The pain rated by patients who experience toxin injection with different needles on different sides of the face confirmed that injection conducted via a finer needle is less painful. Though the sequence of application may have biased the scoring of the pain, in the trial with either a sequence of increasing caliber size from one side to the other or a reverse sequence, all show that the size of needle matters (unpublished study). Usually, most subjects feel minimal pain from the prick of a 30G needle; 31G or 32G needles irritate even less. Topical numbing cream could further alleviate the pricking pain, but this usually is not routinely used before toxin injection because the pain of toxin injection is relatively mild and the procedure is short. Wearing of the needle through trans-stopper toxin aspiration or multiple punctures of the intradermal injection could decrease the needle tip sharpness and cause more pain. Thin-walled needles of the same gauge have smaller needle diameters, performing similarly and less painfully.

Tissue Encountering Pain

Similar to subdermal injection with normal saline, which is quite painful, the pain of toxin injection in tissue is not entirely related to skin puncture but also has to do with the tissue encountering the pharma solution. The pain of drug injection is closely related to the chemical irritancy and pH value of the drug being introduced. That is why a product reconstituted with preserved saline has long been noted to be less painful when the other conditions are kept the same. Sodium bicarbonate and lidocaine have been added to the toxin in reconstitution to decrease the pain of toxin injection without interference in treatment effect. Lactic ringer solution has been used for reconstitution with similar efficacy and less pain. However, clinical efficacy, diffusion profile, and longevity still need to be studied more for compatibility with botulinum toxin as prepared within the guidelines.

The intensity of the pain of tissue encountering toxin fluid is also related to the rate of toxin getting into the tissue. The quick expansion of toxin fluid in tissue usually results in much more and stronger pain.

When comparing the pain of needle insertion with that of toxin infiltration, in the author's experience, the latter usually surpassed the former. While numbing cream alleviates the superficial pricking pain more, that is also the reason that topical anesthesia is not often effective for relieving the pain of toxin injection. Aside from the numbing cream, local infiltration of anesthetics is not recommended as it changes the propensity of toxin spread and tissue thickness. Ice-packing is to be considered for very sensitive patients as it has both numbing and distracting effects.

LENGTH OF NEEDLE

Botulinum toxin that works at the neuromuscular junction theoretically should be delivered as close to the muscle as possible. For insulin syringes, which were originally designed for hypodermal injection away from the face, the dimension of these fixed needles can just approach the level of muscle in most facial zones. But for patients with big masseters or for toxin treatments away from the face, these needles would appear to be too short to reach all the targeted muscle compartments. For injections that need to reach deeper, syringes with detachable needles should be considered. On the other hand, short needles could help control the depth of injection and protect the injector from aberrant insertion and the dangers of false targeting and deep structure damage.

BEVEL OF NEEDLE

Needles introduce bioactive substances to the tissue through their opening, and the outlet of needles is usually oblique and transected, presenting as a bevel. That creates a direction for the outflow. The direction of the flow is meaningful for minimal doses of toxin as these minor differences could be extrapolated into clinical effects, presenting as uneven, asymmetric, and other unpredictable results. For superficial dermal effects, bevels should be kept up with the needle shallowly inserted in at the depth that just immerses the bevel. The direction of needle insertion and beveling should be controlled together to achieve the best symmetry (see Chapter 9). When the injection is to be performed in regions with stratified muscle structure or in slim subjects, needles should be held at an appropriate angle to avoid unnecessary spread and unwanted muscle paralysis.

BIBLIOGRAPHY

Alam M, et al. Effect of needle size on pain perception in patients treated with Botulinum toxin type A injections: A randomized clinical trial. *JAMA Dermatol* 2015;151(11):1194–1199.

Dashtipour K, Chen JJ, Espay AJ, Mari Z, Ondo W. OnabotulinumtoxinA and AbobotulinumtoxinA dose conversion: A systematic literature review. *Mov Disord Clin Pract* 2016;3(2):109–115.

Flanagan T, et al. Size doesn't matter: Needle gauge and injection pain. *Gen Dent* 2007;55(3):216–217.

Flynn TC, et al. Surgical pearl: The use of the Ultra-Fine II short needle 0.3-cc insulin syringe for botulinum toxin injections. *J Am Acad Dermatol* 2002;46(6):931–933.

Foglietti MA, et al. Botulinum toxin therapy: Is syringe type related to cost-effectiveness? *Ann Plast Surg* 2018;80(3):287–289.

Golan S, et al. The association between needle size and waste product and its effect on cost-effectiveness of botulinum toxin injections? *Facial Plast Surg* 2020;36(4):484–486.

Irkoren S, et al. A clinical comparison of EMLA Cream and Ethyl Chloride spray application for pain relief of forehead Botulinum toxin injection. *Ann Plast Surg* 2015;75(3):272–274.

Pickett A, et al. Improving the accuracy of botulinum toxin injections cannot rely on syringe devices. *J Clin Aesthet Dermatol* 2021;14(1):12–13.

Price KM, et al. Needle preference in patients receiving cosmetic botulinum toxin type A. *Dermatol Surg.* 2010;36(1):109–112.

Wambier CG, et al. Flush technique to minimize adverse reactions from syringe lubricant (silicone oil). *J Am Acad Dermatol* 2019;81(6):e169–e171.

8 Achieving Better Symmetry with Aesthetic Toxins

Yates Yen-Yu Chao

CONTENTS

The asymmetry that occurs after toxin modulation is one of the imperfections most often encountered after toxin treatment. It includes but is not restricted to the asymmetry of bilateral contours, dimensions, the position of landmarks, movement patterns, the magnitude of dynamicity, ranges of motion, the homogeneity of remaining muscle activity and muscle strength, and the range, severity, depth, and amount of wrinkles.

The reasons behind these asymmetries include asymmetric injection on a symmetric face, an originally asymmetric face not improved or worsened after toxin treatments, and the multiple minor errors that lead to asymmetric results.

As treatment toxin doses are usually minimal, the delivery process has to be delicate enough to match the subtle difference in doses that are delivered. However, while there are a lot of variables in the process of toxin injection, most of the teaching and training focuses on the number of units and points of injection. Injectors must keep in mind that the activities of muscles to be inhibited by the toxin are usually functionally *normal* and symmetric. The cessation of neuromuscular transmission could not be termed normal, but it is the expected effect if the treatment has been done correctly. However, if any deviation from symmetry occurs because of injection imperfections, it of course would be considered abnormal and the treatment wrong. There are still some patients who continue to be afraid of botulinum toxin simply because it is a toxin. The interruption between the nerve ending and the terminal responding structures is essentially powerful, devastating, and irreversible in the short term. These changes outside of their expectations would horrify them and convince them even more that toxin is dangerous and uncontrollable.

DOI: 10.1201/9781003008132-8

SYMMETRIC ASSUMPTION

Without major asymmetric problems presenting before treatment, all patients should be well photo-documented and considered as symmetric subjects. The toxin should not be delivered asymmetrically in patients without major asymmetry and without pretreatment notification of their asymmetric problems. But in fact, every face, on close inspection, can be found to have some asymmetry. These minimal asymmetries have usually become familiar and are seldom recognized as flaws. These asymmetries should not be specially addressed and tend to present after treatment as well, in a similar pattern to the original asymmetry before treatments. The work of symmetric toxin is more like symmetric inhibition of the target structure activity. However, the intention of symmetric dampening of muscle function could be hampered by some faults, resulting in new asymmetries. There are quite a few points to be emphasized during treatments to ensure the delivery of toxin is in a symmetric pattern. These tips for symmetry include the following:

AIR BUBBLES

Reconstituted toxin fluid within the syringe should present continuously. The flow of the pharma fluid out of the needle is controlled by the hydrostatic pressure via the push of the finger on the plunger. If air gets into the syringe during the drug extraction process, the air that stays between the fluid phases can separate the product and complicate the pressure mechanics and injecting process (Figure 8.1). The pressure delivered via the plunger compresses the mixture of air and fluid. The air inside is more compressible and expandable when compared with the fluid. That pressure, when conveyed to the air between two segments of fluid, compresses the air. This interruption compromises pressure transmission and results in lags and uncertainty in pressure conduction (Figure 8.2). The other segment of fluid then increases in hydrostatic pressure when the air reexpands. The fine movements of the finger for the purpose of fine grid-wise output become much less connected to pressure conduction. It then becomes impossible to achieve precision in dosing..

The imprecision and time-lag of fluid output greatly increase the uncertainty of toxin treatment and leak outside of the tissue. Uncertainty arises as this scenario plays unequally in bilateral corresponding spots. Then asymmetry occurs.

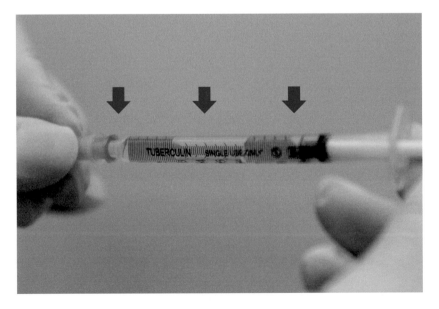

FIGURE 8.1 Because of the tendency to water adhesion, the air existing within the syringe between fluid phases is more difficult to move, to group together, and to smoothly expel out.

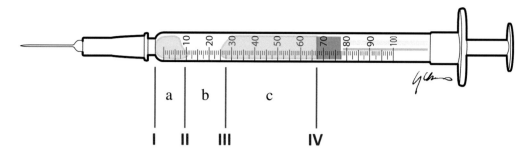

FIGURE 8.2   When air situated between fluid phases (b) is not evacuated completely, the multiple interfaces hinder pressure transmission. Air phases are more compressible and tend to delay the pressure transmission. The reexpansion of air could expel the fluid out after the hand maneuver has stopped and could increase the uncertainty of a proper dosing being administered.

That is why it is so important to extract fluid below the liquid surface, avoiding bubbles and the air-expelling process, during toxin syringe preparation. This is fundamental for precision in injection works.

DIGITALIZED DOSING

Traditional toxin injection techniques involve the delivery of toxin as a simple spatial arrangement in several points with a specific number of units; modern toxin injection techniques adopt more personal variations and individual tailoring. Injection points can vary in number and location between subjects, and the amount of toxin introduced at different points can be different according to the muscle movement patterns. However, in both practices, the main point of symmetric treatment is to deliver exactly the same doses of toxin on both sides of the face. For each side treated with more customized dosing, the arrangement should be repeated for the other side to make sure every change that happens during the treatment procedure is identical from side to side.

INSERTION POINTS

A symmetrical and precise treatment plan, even if it comprises only three or four points each side, should be mirrored identically in corresponding locations. To ensure the work on one side of the face is mirror-symmetrical to the other side, the toxin injection process should be recorded in a digitalized manner, including specified units at specified locations. To repeat the toxin injection to be exactly the same for both sides does not mean simply that (e.g.) the points are all 1 cm away from a landmark, like the lateral canthus; the distance above and below the landmark impacts on treatment effect, too. That means a precise 2D localization for injection points is required for toxin precision. It is even more important for individualized injection ways. As the customized regimes are more varied in spatial arrangement and divergent in dosing among points, it becomes more challenging to repeat them identically on the other side.

For example, toxin treatment for crow's feet usually involves several points of injection arranged in an arc pattern at the lateral margin around the eye. The distance between an injection point and the eye aperture and the distance from the brow – i.e. the exact X- and Y-location, using a landmark (e.g. the lateral canthus) as the reference point – means a lot. Merely controlling the distance from injection point to the canthus without controlling the distance to the brow could result in asymmetric after-treatment brow position; maintaining the distance from the brow without controlling the distance to the canthus axis could leave the remaining periorbital muscle activity and residual wrinkles asymmetric.

INSERTION DEPTH

When comparable points of injection on both sides have been controlled identically in two dimensions (i.e. the dosing and location of the injections are well controlled, being administered symmetrically and equally), we have to further explore the exact depth of needle insertion and to keep the similarity in a 3D pattern. The experience of the author in teaching toxin injection has been that the depth of toxin injection throughout the whole face usually fluctuates and that stable control of needle insertion is extremely difficult. Partly due to their efforts to control the plunger push exactly and to count units, injectors usually are too preoccupied to be aware of the subtle differences in needle depth. Loose tissue lets the needle go in easily, while the needle encounters more resistance in thicker skin. In both circumstances, practitioners could go beyond the expected depth and inject the toxin deeper, but injections of toxin at discrepant depths could result in different clinical effects.

The injection of toxin should be as close to the motor endplates as possible, so the depth of injection should be tailored to match the structural variance (see Chapter 13). Discerning skin thickness is another necessary task for toxin injection procedures. To maintain a certain distance to a certain landmark only controls the spatial arrangement of injection points in two dimensions; the same 2D arrangement but with an additional same-depth regimen advances precision into the third dimension.

POSTURE OF INJECTION

The injector's preference for positioning to one side or the other of the patient has an impact on aesthetic toxin injections. In work requiring symmetry, the posture of injection becomes important because most of the injections proceed via oblique needle insertion. That means the injections are directional. The posture of the injector, the position of the injector relative to the patient, and the posture of the patient can all interfere further with symmetric judgment and practice from side to side. For example, a right-handed injector standing at the right side of a patient injecting toxin in both sides will have the needle inserting into the skin in a different direction and a different angle on the right and on the left. If this injector injects standing at the left side and treating the left face, the direction and angle could be more akin to the right face injection even with the needle in his right hand (Figure 8.3a,b). Right-handed practice accesses the patient differently when approaching the right face at the right side and the left face at the left side, but this can be adjusted.

Strategies to avoid this discrepancy include vertical needle insertion and injecting the patient from behind or in front of the patient.

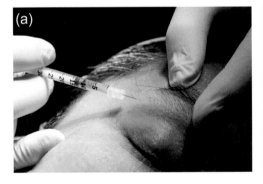 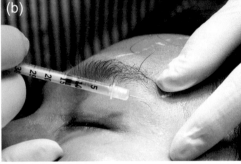

FIGURE 8.3   (a,b) When the practitioner injects both sides of the patient from one side and inserts the needle obliquely, the flow of injectable pharmaceutical is in the direction away from the needle at an angle to the skin surface. That kind of directional flow would not be mirrored symmetrically in comparable regions on either side of the face.

BEVEL DIRECTION

Oblique insertion of a needle delivers the toxin in a certain direction. The bevel of a needle influences the direction in which toxin comes out of the instrument. The direction of the bevel should be controlled more for the purpose of delivering it precisely and symmetrically. In injections via an oblique needle insertion, the bevel should also be adjusted up or down instead of to the side to avoid more complicated aberrant flow.

ANGLE OF NEEDLE

Injection points relative to a surface landmark or anatomical structures have been described well for various aesthetic indications. However, the angle of needle insertion further extends through the skin into the actual point of toxin function. In vertical insertion, toxin is delivered at the same location but flows in the direction of the bevel. In oblique insertion, the toxin effect is a little distance away from the point of insertion, with the distance and depth like the arms of an inserted needle triangle. In near-horizontal insertion, the toxin is delivered toward the surface or toward the superficial structure below.

ASYMMETRIC CONDITIONS

Botulinum toxin can be indicated in patients with asymmetric problems. Sometimes toxin is expected to improve the condition of these asymmetries. Though minimal asymmetry exists in almost every subject, in this section, the discussion concerns pathological or obvious asymmetries.

For problems of static or contour asymmetry that can be improved by toxin modulation, it is more realistic and easier to titrate the doses between sides to approach them more equally. However, for asymmetric dynamic excursions of muscle, it is much more challenging to achieve dynamic symmetry without interfering with static or contour symmetries.

NORMAL STRUCTURAL ASYMMETRY

The span of muscle and pattern of muscle distribution could be different from side to side. Such minor differences can usually be managed with careful assessment and modification during treatments. Aging symptoms can be observed to be more severe on one side because of sleeping postures or sun-exposure environments. These structural rather than functional differences are not recommended to be treated by the functional intervention of toxin except when used for contouring purposes. Masseter asymmetry is not rare because of the habitual preference of unilateral masticatory muscles. Masticatory asymmetry could happen in cases of temporomandibular joint problems, bruxism, or malocclusion. Toxin should be used to help some of these problems, selectively treating part of the muscle, or dosing can be altered to decrease the discrepancy. The same principle is applied also to treat hypertrophic asymmetries of body indications (Figure 8.4a,b).

NORMAL FUNCTIONAL ASYMMETRY

Asymmetric muscle excursion between sides usually results in deviation, unequal movements, or landmark disparity. These minor functional discrepancies can be congenital, developmental, or habitual. Increasing toxin dose in an area with more contraction can usually suppress the hypertonicity to achieve better symmetry.

Functional brow asymmetry is often encountered with the position of the eyebrow or with unequal movements. Toxin correction can be achieved by minimal boosting doses at the more active side or the opposite side on its opponent muscles. Injection points and doses should be judged carefully according to the remaining muscle strength and the extent of the disparity. Practitioners can attain

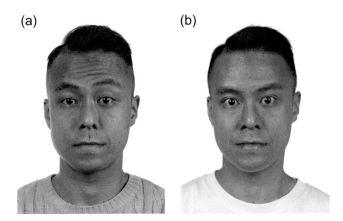

FIGURE 8.4   (a) Asymmetry of the upper face is seen before treatment, including wrinkle orientation, density, depth, brow level, and eye opening. Careful evaluation should be done before toxin treatment to confirm the reasons for these asymmetries. (b) Functional asymmetry can be adjusted via toxin moderation. However, it is not possible and necessary to achieve perfect symmetry through botulinum toxin in view of the structural disparity.

more symmetrical results step by step with minimal dose increments depending on the response to the initial treatment. Injectors should always keep in mind that differential treatment and overdosing of the correcting injection could possibly lead to another asymmetry.

Iatrogenic Asymmetry

Aberrant toxin injection techniques can lead to asymmetric results. This imbalance occurs more after toxin treatment of the upper face or around the eyes than without treatment. When asymmetry happens but the given doses are still low, there still is room for correction and modulation of the remaining muscle activity. More toxin can be added to lessen the asymmetry. If doses for the asymmetry are already high, in some instances, minimal toxin can be carefully applied to the counteracting opponent muscles. The unevenness of toxin distribution can be camouflaged with a touch-up on the gaps in between. However, not every error arising from poor technique can be rescued by more toxin. Because its effect on tissue is only temporary, these faults will disappear, and these patients need to be assured of their full recovery.

Dysfunctional Asymmetry Due to Injury

Damage-related neuromuscular dysfunction leads to impaired muscular activities and will not usually be symmetrical. The reasons behind the damage could be trauma, treatments, or various kind of injury. Toxin has been used to balance these problems of paralysis and dysfunction. However, toxin works by inhibiting neuromuscular function, not restoring it. When the relatively normal side is further paralyzed by botulinum toxin to be compatible with the dysfunctional side, bilateral paralysis may look more symmetrical but may not look normal or be the best result. The larger picture after treatment will be one of increased immobilization. Any attempts to balance these dysfunctional situations must be cautious. Dosing in these treatments is usually empirical. Overdosing could lead to reverse asymmetry and further loss of normal function.

Pathological Asymmetry

Asymmetric neuromuscular dysfunction can be due to pathological reasons. The treatment of pathological dysfunction should be targeted at stopping the progression of the disease and restoring function. Toxin should be reserved for irreversible sequels. The principles for camouflaging these asymmetries are similar to those for traumatic reasons (see section "Dysfunctional Asymmetry Due to Injury" above).

Structural asymmetries due to pathological or traumatic causes should be treated with structural reconstructive procedures. The toxin can be helpful in magnifying the effects of these treatments, including surgery, without replacing their role of structural reconstruction.

COMPENSATIONAL ASYMMETRY

Visible neuromuscular function can be caused by compensatory effects, and these compensations can be asymmetric because they correspond to the underlying reasons being asymmetric. Treatments should be directed toward solving the underlying problem instead of tackling the apparent symptom with toxin. For example, eyebrow position reflects in some cases the compensatory elevation of the frontalis to counteract the drooping of eyelids. The side with more redundant eyelid skin usually has the brow more elevated. Differential surgical trimming of the eyelids with symmetric dosing of forehead toxin is a much more appropriate treatment than differential doses of toxin suppressing the frontalis. The asymmetric toxin can lead to asymmetric frontal motility, worsen the problem of eyelid ptosis, and reveal the underlying eyelid asymmetry.

BIBLIOGRAPHY

Auada Souto MP, et al. An unusual adverse event of botulinum toxin injection in the lower face. *J Cosmet Dermatol* 2021;20(5):1381–1384.

Cabin JA, et al. Botulinum toxin in the management of facial paralysis. *Curr Opin Otolaryngol Head Neck Surg* 2015;23(4):272–280.

Cho YM, et al. Botulinum toxin injection to treat masticatory movement disorder corrected mandibular asymmetry in a growing patient. *J Craniofac Surg* 2019;30(6):1850–1854.

Cooper L, et al. Botulinum toxin treatment for facial palsy: A systematic review. *J Plast Reconstr Aesthet Surg* 2017;70(6):833–841.

Lee SK, et al. Asymmetry and maldistribution of polyacrylamide hydrogel filler in the infraorbital area successfully managed with botulinum toxin a treatment. *Dermatol Surg* 2016;42(12):1395–1397.

Luvisetto S, et al. Botulinum toxin and neuronal regeneration after traumatic injury of central and peripheral nervous system. *Toxins* 2020;12(7):434.

Sneath J, et al. Injecting botulinum toxin at different depths is not effective for the correction of eyebrow asymmetry. *Dermatol Surg* 2015;41(Suppl 1):S82–S87.

Trindade De Almeida AR, et al. Foam during reconstitution does not affect the potency of botulinum toxin type A. *Dermatol Surg* 2003;29(5):530–531.

9 Optimizing Aesthetic Toxin Treatments by Proper Toxin Reconstitution

Jürgen Frevert and Yates Yen-Yu Chao

CONTENTS

TECHNICAL ASPECTS

Jürgen Frevert

RECONSTITUTION PROCEDURE

All botulinum toxin products are reconstituted with preservative-free 0.9% sodium chloride to establish a solution with physiological osmolality according to the product information. The products have different appearance due to the drying process: onabotulinumtoxin appears as a thin film on the bottom of the vial, and abobotulinumtoxin and incobotulinumtoxin as freeze-dried powder (lyophilisates) forming a fluffy cake. The reconstitution procedure therefore differs from product to product. Incobotulinumtoxin has to be prepared by swirling and inverting/flipping the vial after the injection of saline through the rubber stopper. When the vial is not inverted, part of the product at the rubber stopper might get lost (Carey 2014). The products dissolve immediately; vigorous shaking is not necessary, although it does not affect the potency as the neurotoxin is not a labile substance (Kazim & Black 2008).

RECONSTITUTION AND TOXIN CONCENTRATION

The reconstitution volume can range between 0.5 mL and 10 mL depending on the product, the therapeutic requirements and the dosage (50 U, 100 U or 200 U, incobotulinumtoxin or onabotulinumtoxin, and 300 U or 500 u of abobotulinumtoxin). This allows the preparation of 1U–40 U per 0.1 mL. The reconstitution volume determines the concentration of the product and the injection volume and affects the spread.

DOI: 10.1201/9781003008132-9

67

Reconstitution and Injection Pain

The injection of products reconstituted with saline as recommended can cause injection-site pain ("pricking"). It can be demonstrated that the pain results from the low pH of the saline (the products are not buffered) (Dressler et al. 2016). The authors reconstituted off label with a buffered solution (Ringer acetate) and found the same efficacy, but no injection-site pain was reported by the patients. Some physicians reconstitute off label with antibacterial saline containing benzoyl alcohol. It was reported that injection-site pain was also reduced with this solution with no reduction of efficacy (Alam et al. 2002), suggesting that the pH of this diluent is also neutral. Reconstitution with lidocaine (off label) can also reduce injection-site pain (Güleç 2012, Vadoud-Seyedi & Simonart 2007).

Stability of Reconstituted Toxin

The stability of the reconstituted products is different from that of the dried products. Unreconstituted incobotulinum can be stored at room temperature (<25°C), whereas abobotulinumtoxin and onabotulinumtoxin have to be stored at 2–8°C in the refrigerator. This also refutes the claim that the complexing proteins contained in both Ona and Abo would be required for stability. The reason for the high stability of Inco might be due to its optimized formulation and/or purity, i.e. that it is devoid of impurities which may affect stability. All reconstituted products must be stored at 2–8° C and have to be used within 24 hours according to the license. The reason for this is that, bacteria could grow in the reconstituted vial. If the product is reconstituted under strict sterile conditions, the stability is substantially longer, at least for Inco. The reconstituted Inco was stored at room temperature for 14 days and then analyzed in a head-to-head trial (glabellar lines) with freshly reconstituted Inco, which demonstrated no decrease in efficacy (Soares et al. 2015).

Dilution and Toxin Spread

Spread describes the distribution of molecules from the injection site and is governed by e.g. injection technique, volume of injection, needle size, angle of needle, and force of injection. In contrast, *diffusion* is a physical term and indicates the passive movement of neurotoxin along a concentration gradient in a liquid. According to Fick's law, molecules with a higher molecular weight will diffuse more slowly than molecules with a lower molecular weight. Because adverse events are caused by the movement of botulinum toxin molecules into muscles not to be treated, it was hypothesized that Inco with pure 150 kD neurotoxin would diffuse faster than the 900 kD complex. However, by analyzing the protein species in reconstituted vials, it was found that in Ona, the neurotoxin was dissociated from the complexing proteins (only 15% of the neurotoxin was bound in a small complex). The complexes in abobotulinumtoxin were completely dissociated. This result demonstrates that the spread of the 150 kD neurotoxin is unaffected by the complexing proteins (Eisele et al. 2011) (Figure 9.1). Moreover, the dissociation is a prerequisite for bioactivity at the nerve, since the complex-bound neurotoxin cannot bind to its receptors because the binding domain is shielded by one of the complexing proteins so that the binding is blocked (Gu et al. 2012). In conclusion, when injected in an equipotent dose, all products should show the same spreading behavior. This was demonstrated in mice when Abo, Ona, and Inco were injected in comparable doses (Carli et al. 2009). A split phase study confirmed this result: the products were injected in comparable doses and identical volumes into the frontalis muscle, and the area of anhydrosis was determined. There was no difference in the area of anhydrosis when Inco and Ona were compared; however, the area caused by Abo was larger. This could be the result of a higher number of active neurotoxin molecules being injected when applying a dose ratio of 1:2.5. This would also explain the observation that Abo "diffuses more" than the other products. The neurotoxin in Abo spreads in a similar fashion to the neurotoxins of the other products because it is the same protein – the larger area of anhydrosis is only a reflection of the higher dose. It was hypothesized that the very low

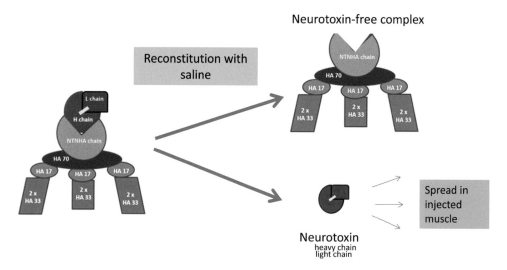

FIGURE 9.1 Dissociation of the botulinum complex. After reconstitution, the complex dissociates. The neurotoxin spreads in the injected tissue, unaffected by the complexing proteins.

amount of serum albumin in abobotulinumtoxin (0.125 mg/vial) might be responsible for the faster spread of Abo. The concentration of human serum albumin in the interstitial fluid is approximately 60 mg/mL (Kutschenko et al. 2019), substantially higher than the concentration in the products. After injection, the neurotoxin in all products would immediately be taken to the level of the much higher HSA concentration in the tissue.

The spread of the neurotoxin molecules within the tissue is mainly determined by the dose and by the volume of injection. A higher volume leads to more spread. There is an optimal injection volume with an optimal dose that depends on the size of the muscle. A small muscle would be effectively treated with a low volume (high concentration) injected close to the neuromuscular junctions. A more voluminous muscle requires a larger volume or a higher number of injections, which would be more favorable for reaching all neuromuscular junctions. The effect of a higher solution should be not overestimated: an injection of 5 U in 0.25 mL on one side of the forehead and in 0.025 mL on the other side resulted in a 50% larger area when injected with a 5-fold higher volume (Hsu et al. 2004). This is in keeping with early studies in which it was found that a 10-fold higher injection volume in the treatment of glabellar lines did not show any decrease in effect and, most importantly, no increase in side effects (Carruthers et al. [0.1 vs 1.0 mL]). A different result was shown when two different volumes were injected into the forehead (6 U of Abo in 0.1 or 0.3 mL). The higher injection volume produced an area of wrinkle reduction about 67% greater than the concentrated dose (0.1 mL). But there was substantial variation between the patients due to e.g. differences in the bulk of muscle and dynamic movement of muscle.

Increasing the dose of several botulinum toxin products from 1 U in 0.01 mL to 5 U in 0.05 mL (both dose and volume were increased) led to an increase in the mean area of anhydrosis to about 300% (Costa et al. 2012). Although the product was injected into the skin and not into the muscle, it can be assumed that an increase of dose and the volume by a factor of 5 increases the spread substantially. In clinical practice, the dose and injection volume are certainly not increased by such a high factor; consequently there seems to be flexibility for the physician in terms of choosing an appropriate injection volume. It is more important to inject close to the neuromuscular junctions to achieve an optimal effect and a long duration (resulting in optimal "loading" of the nerve terminals with the light chain of the neurotoxin). On the other hand, it would be possible to increase the dose by keeping the volume low (high concentration) in order to prolong the duration without sacrificing safety.

CLINICAL IMPLICATIONS

Yates Yen-Yu Chao

CLINICAL PRACTICE OF TOXIN RECONSTITUTION

The process of toxin manufacturing and how the toxin is reconstituted can have an impact on the final amount of toxin available for clinical use, because lyophilized products have botulinum toxin as fluffy coats that also stick to the stopper. Without adequate swirling or inversion, toxin molecules may be separated out, resulting in a lower toxin concentration. This problem can be more prominent in Inco; although Abo is manufactured by a similar process, it is sold in a much smaller vial and the reconstitution often fills the vial. Inco also has stoppers that sequestrate more liquid inside (Figure 9.2). If the stopper is not removed from the vial, injectors could leave some active ingredients behind or inject less when the injection quantity is counted by vial (like armpit or calf). Inco has more protein (human serum albumin) contents, albeit with no complexing protein. Protein substances foam upon flushing (Figure 9.3a); foam interferes with the normal distribution of active molecules. Reconstitution should have the saline infusion needle adhere to the bottle wall and avoid a quick flush (Figure 9.3b,c). Drug extraction should be delayed until the foam has resolved, to ensure the pharma protein is in the right concentration.

RECONSTITUTION AND INJECTION PAIN

The pain of a toxin injection can be divided into the pain of needle prick and the pain of in vivo fluid expansion. The pain of toxin in tissue is pH related and can be relieved somewhat by using preserved saline or adding lidocaine or sodium bicarbonate without diminishing the therapeutic toxin effect.

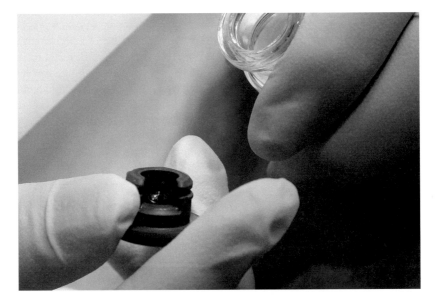

FIGURE 9.2   Adhesion tendency of a fluid retains fluid in dead spaces. The vial stopper "grotto" plays this role, and residual toxin fluid can be often found when toxin is thought to have run out and the stopper is removed. When toxin dosing is counted by vial – for example, in body indications – the clinical effect could be misunderstood as inferior because of incomplete consumption.

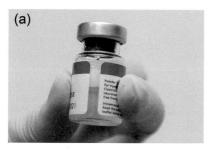 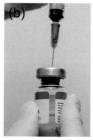 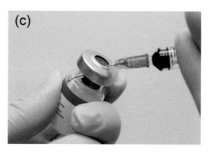

FIGURE 9.3 A thick layer of foam (a) can be visible when the reconstitution proceeds as a rapid flush of saline through a free-hanging needle (b). That is unique and most prominent for incobotulinum toxin. The reconstitution needle should adhere to the vial wall, importing saline with flow following the vial wall (c).

DILUTION AND TOXIN SPREAD

Toxin spread has long been discussed for the purpose of determining the exact range of blocks for best practice. Fick's law is usually given as the reason for the movement of active toxin molecules, describing the movement driven by a concentration gradient, and concentration level is closely related to the volume of saline added during reconstitution. However, the spread of toxin in tissue is not pure diffusion. As most of the judgment of toxin diffusion is done on the forehead by measuring the diameter of anhidrosis after toxin injection, more discussion on diffusion will be included in Chapter 16.

BIBLIOGRAPHY

Abbasi NR, et al. A small study of the relationship between Abobotulinum toxin A concentration and forehead wrinkle reduction. *Arch Dermatol* 2012;148(1):119–121.

Alam M, et al. Pain associated with injection of botulinum A exotoxin reconstituted using isotonic sodium chloride with and without preservative: A double-blind, randomized controlled trial. *Arch Dermatol* 2002;138:510–514.

Botox (Allergan), *Summary of product characteristics*, United Kingdom, 2019.

Carey WD. Incorrect reconstitution of IncobotulinumtoxinA leads to loss of neurotoxin. *J Drugs Dermatol* 2014;13:735–738.

Carli L, et al. Assay of diffusion of different botulinum neurotoxin type A formulations injected in the mouse leg. *Muscle Nerve* 2009;40:374–380.

Costa A, et al. Comparative study of the diffusion of five botulinum toxins type-A in five dosages of use: Are there differences amongst the commercially-available products? *Dermatol Online J* 2012;18:2.

Dover JS, et al. Botulinum toxin in aesthetic medicine: Myths and realities. *Dermatol Surg* 2018;44(2):249–260.

Dressler D, et al. Reconstituting botulinum toxin drugs: Shaking, stirring or what? *J Neural Transm (Vienna)* 2016;123(5):523–525.

Dressler D, et al. Botulinum toxin therapy: Reduction of injection site pain by pH normalisation. *J Neural Transm* 2016;123(5):527–531.

Dysport (Ipsen), *Summary of product characteristics*, United Kingdom, 2018.

Eisele KH, et al. Studies on the dissociation of botulinum neurotoxin type A complexes. *Toxicon* 2011;57:555–565.

Grein S, et al. Stability of botulinum neurotoxin type A, devoid of complexing proteins. *The Botulinum J* 2011;2:49–58.

Güleç AT. Dilution of botulinum toxin A in lidocaine vs. in normal saline for the treatment of primary axillary hyperhidrosis: A double-blind, randomized, comparative preliminary study. *J Eur Acad Dermatol Venereol* 2012;26(3):314–318.

Gu S, et al. Botulinum neurotoxin is shielded by NTNHA in an interlocked complex. *Science* 2012; 335:977–981.

Hexsel D, et al. A randomized pilot study comparing the action halos of two commercial preparations of botulinum toxin type A. *Dermatol Surg* 2008;34:52–59.

Hsu TS, et al. Effect of volume and concentration on the diffusion of botulinum exotoxin A. *Arch Dermatol* 2004;140:1351–1354.

Kazim NA, Black EH. Botox: Shaken, not stirred. *Ophthalmic Plast Reconstr Surg* 2008;24(1):10–12.

Kerscher M, et al. Comparison of the spread of three botulinum toxin type A preparations. *Arch Dermatol Res* 2012;304:155–161.

Kutschenko A, et al. The role of human serum albumin and neurotoxin associated proteins in the formulation of BoNT/A products. *Toxicon* 2019;168:158–163.

Pickett A. Dysport: Pharmacological properties and factors that influence toxin action. *Toxicon* 2009;54:683–689.

Ramirez-Castaneda J, et al. Diffusion, spread, and migration of botulinum toxin. *Mov Disord* 2013;28(13):1775–1783.

Soares DJ, et al. Impact of postreconstitution room temperature storage on the efficacy of incobotulinumtoxinA treatment of dynamic lateral canthus lines. *Dermatol Surg* 2015;41:712–717.

Vadoud-Seyedi J, et al. Treatment of axillary hyperhidrosis with botulinum toxin type A reconstituted in lidocaine or in normal saline: A randomized, side-by-side, double-blind study. *Br J Dermatol* 2007;156:986–989.

Trindade de Almeida AR, et al. Pilot study comparing the diffusion of two formulations of botulinum toxin type A in patients with forehead hyperhidrosis. *Dermatol Surg* 2007;33 Spec No.:S37–S43.

Xeomin (Merz), *Summary of product characteristics*, United Kingdom, 2020.

10 The Initial Judgment and Repeating and Modifying Aesthetic Toxin Treatments

Yates Yen-Yu Chao

CONTENTS

Aesthetic toxin treatments usually have clinical effects lasting for 4–6 months. Patients who want to maintain the toxin's effects have to repeat the treatment periodically. How a successful treatment can be continued in successive sessions depends on how these treatment details are repeated. As minimal alterations to toxin administration could result in exponential effects, aesthetic treatments with toxin should not fluctuate in the pattern of injection or in individual and relative dosing. In other words, the pattern, extent, and degree of inhibition have to be reproducible. Good and appropriate effects of modulation should be maintained while lessons also should be learned from each treatment session, helping to modify the regimen of the next injection.

It is interesting and apparent that the protocols of aesthetic toxin treatment 20 years ago generally used doses higher than in modern practice, and the toxin doses per injection spot are also higher. With the evolution of aesthetic medical practice and a better understanding of facial structure anatomy, the traditional and 3-point or 4-point technique that appears simple has been refined into more versified individual regimens. The grid-wise pushing on standard points appears simple but is actually highly dependent on context. To repeat a successful toxin treatment or refine a well-conducted procedure requires professional recording of the treatment details and correct reading of the clinical responses. However, starting treatment in a new patient who has never previously been treated for a specific problem requires more expertise on the toxin and related physiology. The initial correct decision has a great impact on future re-treatments. When a patient has already experienced toxin treatments somewhere else and comes to you, that patient could feel the effects and know the differences. The traditional protocols of aesthetic toxin use may not be the best way to dispense toxin molecules, but they are a model from which you can develop and refine personal skills.

DOI: 10.1201/9781003008132-10

THE INITIAL JUDGMENT

Every patient has his or her problems and needs their toxin treatment administered differently. The most important factor in determining a successful aesthetic toxin treatment is the assessment that helps to form a sensible treatment plan. A complete assessment of the patient includes visual observation and hand palpation. Instrumental examinations, like ultrasound, can provide additional information.

VISUAL EVALUATION

The appearance of the target tissue for botulinum toxin injection can be very informative. Practitioners should observe the candidates from the beginning of the consultation. Normal daily activities like smiling and speaking demonstrate most about the normal excursion pattern of the mimetic muscles. In different facial expressions, visible information about personal muscle synergism is revealed (Figure 10.1a,b). The activity of muscles can be observed through related structural movements. The extent of motion also suggests the range of distribution of the muscle fibers (Figure 10.2).

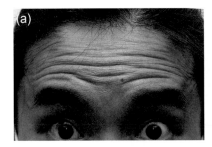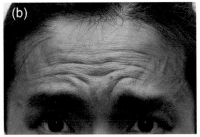

FIGURE 10.1   Both (a) in the movement raising the brow and (b) in the movement of frowning, the frontalis muscle exercises throughout the whole process. However, frontalis activity is limited to the central lower region that synergizes with the frowning corrugator.

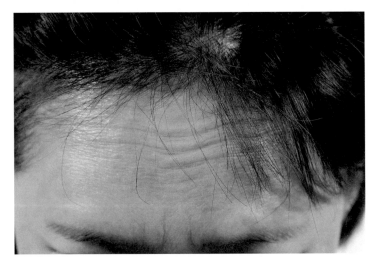

FIGURE 10.2   In this patient, frontalis muscle activity can be detected through visual observation. Both lower lateral parts of the forehead appear relatively calm, and the left side contracts more forcefully than the right side.

Injectors should collect a range of information, including skin thickness (Figure 10.3), skin quality, and skin conditions including seborrhea, telangiectasia, comedones, pimples, active infection, and other inflammatory conditions. Some patients may have contour or quality changes indicating recent or previous treatments that could interfere with toxin injection. Injectors should also recognize innate or iatrogenic problems that could be magnified or worsened after the onset of the toxin effect, such as partial paralysis and structural asymmetries (Figure 10.4a,b,c). All these complicating problems should be explained clearly to patients before treatment and documented thoroughly as a medical record. The previous history of toxin use — including the brand, approximate doses, expense, positive and negative effects, duration of effects, satisfaction, and detailed treatment areas

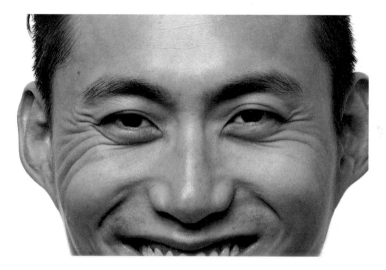

FIGURE 10.3 Through visual observation, the skin folds that form during muscle exercise hint at the skin thickness. The folding of skin is like a sandwich with the epidermis forming both surfaces; the upper lateral canthal skin is thinner than the lower.

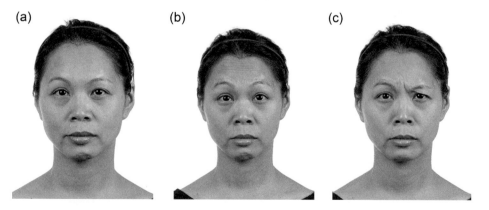

(a)   (b)   (c)

FIGURE 10.4 (a) The pre-treatment photo shows a largely symmetrical face with the resting right eyebrow a little higher and the right nasolabial fold a little blunter. (b) The movement raising the brow is relatively symmetrical with the right side frontal lines pulled a little higher. Eyebrow level appears more symmetrical in full frontal contraction than in the resting state. (c) However, the movement of the frown is almost absent on the right side.

- should also be collected for better judgment. Information about any previous fillers, threads, prosthesis, grafts, previous surgeries, and ongoing procedures or routine skin care should be acquired as well.

More careful observation can also find subtle variations in tiny muscle movements, the vector, tonic contraction, partial accentuation, etc. The activity of the opponent muscles, muscular compensation, and underlying tissue laxity are also important factors for the toxin plan.

COMMUNICATION

In addition to history taking, injectors should be aware of the expectations and motivation of the subjects for the treatment, which helps a lot in decision making concerning the range and dosing of toxin use. The initial symptoms of toxin resistance can sometimes be detected through a careful review of history.

PALPATION

Much of the above information acquired by history taking and visual observation can be further verified by hand palpation. Injectors can use touching the treatment areas to understand more about the skin and its quality, laxity, or thickness (Figure 10.5a,b) and about muscle conditions and their basic tone, thickness, volume (Figure 10.6), distribution, muscular activity, insertion points, superficial tethering fibers (Figure 10.7), strength of motion, synergism, and depth of movement.

Hand palpation is also valuable for the examination of early results when patients return, for detection of a possible incomplete block, and for better understanding of the toxin effect (Figures 10.8, 10.9) and the quality of the treatment. Early resistant cases are usually more detectable at this stage through subtle deterioration in clinical effects; the detection of slight incompleteness cannot rely only on visual observation.

RECORDING AND POSTTREATMENT EVALUATION

A detailed recording of treatment specifications is important for reproducing the desired toxin effects or further improvement in consequent treatment courses. Especially for toxin treatments, one of the key ways to show professionalism is to produce the same result reliably every time patients resume their treatments. A well-kept and complete record helps clinicians improve their expertise in making decisions and forming a treatment plan.

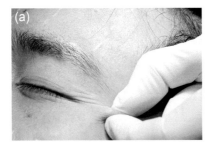 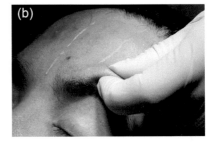

FIGURE 10.5 Skin thickness is well understood to be thinner (a) in the periorbital region than (b) on the forehead. However, measuring the exact thickness by palpation can help with judging the proper depth of needle insertion.

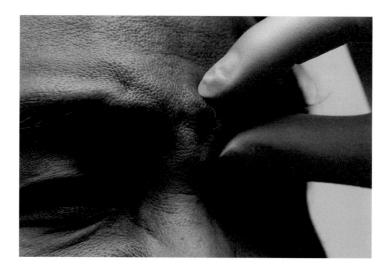

FIGURE 10.6 Muscle volume and distribution can vary from patient to patient. Correct evaluation helps decide the proper treatment dose.

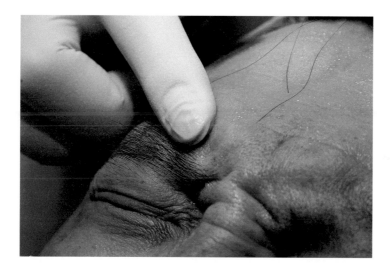

FIGURE 10.7 Facial muscles have more complex interdigitation and connection with other muscles and the skin. The mobility, connection, and restriction of structures can be further recognized through palpable evaluation.

REPEATING TREATMENTS

Aesthetic toxin treatments are popular and have become a recurrent routine for most toxin patients. Quality control is mandatory for practitioners to enable them to offer them as a sustainable business. Even a minor change in point dosage and the arrangement of injecting points could result in changes that weren't anticipated. Any progress or decline can soon be detected by patients, and they perhaps know the difference better than the injector can. Patients will always appreciate the expertise of a professional who can offer precision treatment, resulting in a steady improvement. Since toxin has to be reapplied every 4–6 months, it is embarrassing for the patient to have a face that keeps changing after a period of several months.

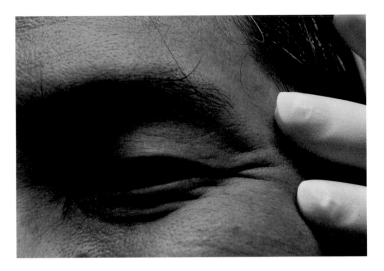

FIGURE 10.8   The range of wrinkles is not actually the range of the muscle. Lines of folding can be the rippling of skin next to the skin sequestration. Hand evaluation is valuable to help understand the underlying muscle activity.

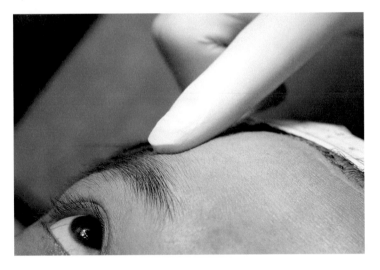

FIGURE 10.9   Residual muscle activity can be present even though there is no visible wrinkle after the treatment, which shows the difference between complete toxin coverage and clinical efficacy.

TREATMENT MAPS OF DOSING AND DEPTH

Before toxin injection can become a personal ongoing program, treatment depth, doses, and points of injection should be well documented for further reference so that any suboptimal results can be tracked and modifications can be made, based on the original plan.

OTHER TREATMENT NOTES

It is important to document clearly by photography and description the problem that the patient wishes to be treated and the associated concerns of the patient, including the pretreatment conditions, asymmetry, synergism, etc.; facial dynamicity itself is transitory, disappearing, and changing very rapidly. These problems can be omitted or masked after the treatment. The problems of a patient change along with the aging process. The many choices of aesthetic intervention nowadays that could change the targets of toxin should be well recorded, too. These records are also valuable for better understanding the efficacy and longevity of the treatments.

MODIFICATION OF TREATMENT PLAN

To keep the treatment results stable, a regimen with satisfactory results and good responses should be reproduced precisely in an ongoing program. But when conditions change, such as through aging, additional surgeries or fillers, weight loss or gain, or the accumulation of treatment effects, how should practitioners adjust their treatment plans?

For most dynamic wrinkle–associated mimetic muscle movements, similar doses of injection are needed if similar effects are expected. But for problems of contouring that involve disuse atrophy, clinical effects usually last longer and treatment doses can be lessened after repeated treatments. Weight gain and training exercises of the treating muscles may have an impact on these contouring toxin treatments, offsetting their clinical effects. Injectable fillers can change structural geometry and the layering relationship, which should be taken into consideration when the toxin is to be applied over or together.

Aging-related sagging and drooping changes the pattern and severity of wrinkles, opponent muscle relationship, and facial dynamicity. Toxin doses are usually expected to be increased upon these changes; however, these concomitant aging symptoms can be better addressed with more appropriate modalities than the continued increment of toxin doses. The usual practice of toxin lifting procedures combats sagging problems through the effect of counteracting elevator muscles. Hyperactive compensatory elevator muscles are not the best and most pathognomonic resolution for tissue laxity or structural sagging.

In practice, injectable fillers and cosmetic surgical procedures are often combined with botulinum toxin injections. For patients who have additional foreign volume within the tissue, toxin doses and treatment patterns would need to be modified to avoid aggregating the superficially deposited foreign substances. Some errors in filler treatment could be helped by minimal doses of toxin to mask the problems of uneven distribution, focal filler accumulation, wrong layering of injections, and filler-related poor contours. Surgeries may change structural tissue planes. The depth of toxin injection should be modified in surgical patients as well. Tissue trimming surgeries solve the problem of tissue redundancy, allowing more flexible toxin administration. Toxin conversely helps these surgeries to relieve the muscles, facilitating wound healing, and to camouflage surgical imperfections.

BIBLIOGRAPHY

de Maio M, et al. Facial assessment and injection guide for botulinum toxin and injectable hyaluronic acid fillers: Focus on the upper face. *Plast Reconstr Surg* 2017;140(2):265e–276e.

de Maio M, et al. Facial assessment and injection guide for botulinum toxin and injectable hyaluronic acid fillers: Focus on the lower face. *Plast Reconstr Surg* 2017;140(3):393e–404e.

Farolch-Prats L, et al. Facial contouring by using dermal fillers and botulinum toxin a: A practical approach. *Aesthetic Plast Surg* 2019;43(3):793–802.

Flynn TC. Botulinum toxin: Examining duration of effect in facial aesthetic applications. *Am J Clin Dermatol* 2010;11(3):183–199.

Glogau R, et al. Assessment of botulinum toxin aesthetic outcomes: Clinical study vs real-world practice. *JAMA Dermatol* 2015;151(11):1177–1178.

Hexsel D, et al. Long-term cumulative effects of repeated botulinum toxin type A injections on brow position. *Dermatol Surg* 2020;46(9):1252–1254.

Nestor M. Key parameters for the use of abobotulinumtoxina in aesthetics: Onset and duration. *Aesthet Surg J* 2017;37(suppl_1):S20–S31.

Weinkle SH, et al. Impact of comprehensive, minimally invasive, multimodal aesthetic treatment on satisfaction with facial appearance: The HARMONY study. *Aesthet Surg J* 2018;38(5):540–556.

11 Anatomical Considerations to Improve Aesthetic Treatments Using Neuromodulators

Nicholas Moellhoff and Sebastian Cotofana

CONTENTS

INTRODUCTION

The face is composed of complex and interwoven anatomical structures, allowing for versatile facial expressions, the display of emotion, communication, food intake, and digestion. Morphological changes in the facial skeleton and soft tissue layers over time, caused by multifactorial processes, lead to facial aging (Cotofana et al. 2016). Knowledge of anatomy and the changes in the soft tissue constitution underlying the process of aging is the key to performing safe and effective treatments, including neuromodulator injections to ameliorate facial rhytids.

Dynamic facial lines reflect the response of the skin surface to a contraction of the underlying musculature. Facial muscles can be attached directly to the overlying skin, allowing for precise facial expression, for example in the eyebrow or periorbital region, or they can exert an indirect effect transmitted by layers of fascia, as is the case in the forehead (Ingallina et al. 2022). In the mid-face, the muscles of facial expression are connected to the skin more loosely, by a three-dimensional fascial network composed of elastic fibers, fat lobules, and connective tissue fibers, referred to as the superficial musculo-aponeurotic system (SMAS) (Sandulescu et al. 2019). Depending on the fiber orientation, muscles can exert several movement axes, including horizontal or vertical contraction patterns or radiating in a peripherally orientated fashion.

DOI: 10.1201/9781003008132-11

Neurotoxins cause muscle paralysis by inhibiting the release of acetylcholine at the neuromuscular junction (Small 2014). Several factors impact the effect of neurotoxin injections, including dosage, volume, depth of injection, and anatomic region, as well as the anatomic fascial layers penetrated (Swift et al. 2022). The anatomy of the facial muscles is highly variable between individuals. Aesthetic outcomes are therefore dependent on precise patient evaluation prior to injection. Both dynamic contraction patterns and muscle fiber orientation, as well as static facial lines, should be assessed to determine the most suitable injection points. While adverse events are not observed frequently, and their duration is limited by the effectiveness of the toxin, they can cause dissatisfaction and can disturb the treated patient (Ahsanuddin et al. 2021). Adverse events are often the consequence of affecting muscles which were not the primary target of injection. In-depth understanding of the underlying musculature with its movement axes is therefore crucial to predict outcomes and to avoid collateral damage.

The following chapter elaborates on the formation of facial wrinkles based on the underlying muscles of facial expression and other common aesthetic indications and illustrates the clinically relevant anatomy for the neuromodulator treatment of different regions.

PERIORBITAL REGION

The periorbital region is of central importance during social interaction. It plays a role in nonverbal communication and displays a large set of emotions, including sadness, tiredness, anger, or surprise. The fascial layered arrangement of the periorbital region is composed of eight distinct anatomical layers:

Layer 1: Skin
Layer 2: Subcutaneous fat
Layer 3: Suprafrontalis fascia/orbicularis retaining ligament
Layer 4: Frontalis muscle/orbicularis oculi muscle
Layer 5: Retro-orbicularis oculi fat (ROOF)
Layer 6: Dense fascia in continuation of the subfrontalis fascia
Layer 7: Preperiosteal fat
Layer 8: Periosteum

The subcutaneous architecture of the eyebrow and glabella enables precise and accurate skin movement. Here, muscle fibers, connective tissue, and subdermal fat are strongly intertwined and adherent to the overlying skin without forming a separate subcutaneous gliding plane which could potentially mask muscle movement (Sykes et al. 2015). Furthermore, the eyebrow has no direct attachment to the underlying bony supraorbital rim, allowing for high and versatile mobility upon contraction of the periorbital musculature. A further prerequisite for the high functionality of the periorbital region is the unique constitution of the periorbital musculature, which is made up of four muscles –the procerus, the corrugator supercilii, the orbicularis oculi, and the frontalis muscle – which all fuse with the skin at the level of the hairy eyebrow (Figure 11.1). However, the muscles of the periorbital region cannot be regarded solely as individual entities as they are interconnected and act as a biomechanical unit, exerting combined effects on the overlying skin of the brow and the glabella. Collectively, they are also referred to as the orbicularis oculi muscle complex.

The orbicularis oculi muscle is located strictly subdermal with contact to the bone and ligaments at the cranial aspect of the tear trough, the tear trough ligament, and the medial canthal ligament. The procerus and corrugator supercilii muscles each have distinct bony origins (Figure 11.2). The origin of the procerus muscle is located at the nasal bone at the root of the nose in the midline and the paramedian plane, and it inserts into the skin of the glabella at the level of the upper margin of the hairy eyebrow. The origin of the corrugator supercilii muscle is the superciliary arch of the frontal bone in the paramedian plane. It inserts the skin in the middle third of the eyebrow. The

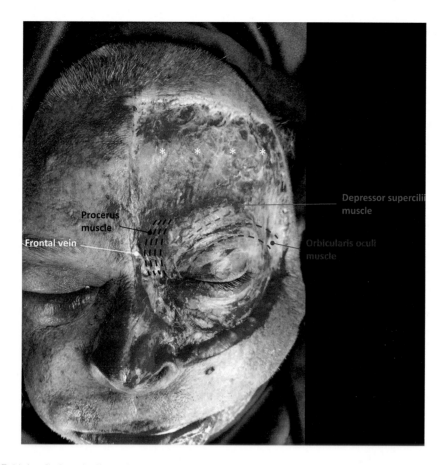

FIGURE 11.1 Cadaveric dissection of the left upper face. The frontalis muscle (*) extends over the forehead with muscle fibers investing into the orbicularis oculi (in the lateral, middle, and medial third of the eyebrow), corrugator supercilii (in the middle third of the eyebrow), and procerus muscle (in the midline) at a horizontal level corresponding to the upper margin of the hairy eyebrow.

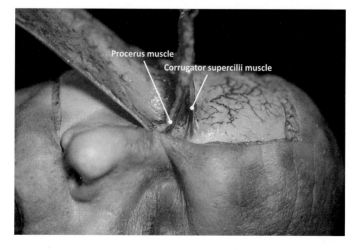

FIGURE 11.2 Cadaveric dissection of the glabella region. Note the bony origin of the procerus and corrugator supercilii muscle.

frontalis muscle has no bony connection but is enveloped by two fasciae extending from the galea aponeurotica. While it extends over the forehead, its muscle fibers invest into the orbicularis oculi (in the lateral, middle, and medial third of the eyebrow), corrugator supercilii (in the middle third of the eyebrow), and procerus muscle (in the midline) at a horizontal level, corresponding to the upper margin of the hairy eyebrow (Figure 11.1).

Importantly, the middle third of the eyebrow is primarily pulled medially by the dermal insertion of the corrugator supercilii muscle, while the medial third of the eyebrow responds via muscular connections to the medial orbicularis oculi (also referred to as the depressor supercilii muscle) and lateral parts of the procerus muscle (depression of the medial brow). The frontalis muscle, on the other hand, is the main eyebrow elevator. Laterally, the orbicularis oculi muscle acts as a depressor of the lateral brow.

Given the complexity of this anatomical region, prior to performing injection of neuromodulators to ameliorate glabella frown lines or for brow shape adjustments, practitioners should have advanced knowledge of the anatomic location and the complex interplay between the individual periorbital muscles to ensure effectiveness, efficiency, and safety and to tailor injection plans to the individual patient.

GLABELLA FROWN LINES

Glabella lines result from contraction of the corrugator supercilii, the orbicularis oculi (depressor supercilii) and the procerus muscle. Vertical and horizontal glabellar lines are differentiated, depending on the axis of movement. As a rule of principle, the orientation of the rhytids is perpendicular to the muscle fascicle contraction. Thus, horizontal lines are caused by procerus muscle contraction, while vertical lines are predominantly caused by contraction of the corrugator supercilii muscle (pulling horizontally on the skin of the middle eyebrow), in combination with contraction of the medial component of the orbicularis oculi muscle, with lateral fibers of the procerus muscle also contributing to their formation.

The eyebrow position is at a balance between antagonistic muscle groups, i.e. the depressors and elevators of the brow. Disturbing this equilibrium, i.e. by injecting neuromodulators to reduce dynamic glabella frown lines, will paralyze the targeted muscle or muscle groups, therefore ultimately also affecting eyebrow position. The aim should be to target the individual muscles responsible for formation of the frown lines, and to ensure precise product placement to prevent over- or undertreatment or unintended muscle relaxation due to product diffusion.

Hence, a 3-point injection technique for treating the glabella was proposed recently, targeting the procerus and the corrugator supercilii muscles exclusively at their respective bony origin (Cotofana et al. 2021). Injecting deeply, in contact with the bone, will distribute the product efficiently into the muscle belly, resulting in prompt onset of relaxation, while reducing collateral damage at the same time. To target the origin of the corrugator muscle, the injector should place the needle 1–2 mm medial and inferior to the medial end of the noncontracted hairy eyebrow, and apply the product in contact with the bone (Cotofana et al. 2021). The origin of the procerus muscle is injected at the midline in the level of a connecting line between the left and right medial canthal ligaments (Cotofana et al. 2021). Additional subdermal injection points may be placed within the medial third of the eyebrow should a muscular contraction at the upper margin of the hairy eyebrow be visible, in order to target the medial parts of the orbicularis oculi muscle (depressor supercilii).

LATERAL CANTHAL LINES

Lateral canthal lines, also referred to as crow's feet, result from contraction of the lateral fibers of the orbicularis oculi muscle. As the subdermal muscle fiber orientation is arranged in a circular way around the bony orbit, the rhytids that result after contraction radiate in a peripherally orientated fashion. The constitution of the skin and subcutaneous fat layer determines the depth of the rhytids, while the extension of the underlying orbicularis oculi muscle determines the length. Subdermal injection of neurotoxin may reduce the severity of these rhytids. Weakening of the muscle also causes elevation of the tail of the eyebrow, as once again the balance between the depressor (orbicularis oculi muscle) and elevator (frontalis muscle) of the brow is shifted.

COMMON ADVERSE EVENTS WHEN TREATING THE PERIORBITAL REGION

- *Eyebrow ptosis*
  The corrugator supercilii muscle is often injected at its dermal insertion at the upper border of the middle eyebrow. Placement of neuromodulator injections above the eyebrow can cause eyebrow ptosis due to relaxation of the frontalis muscle, which is responsible for eyebrow elevation. In addition, injecting the procerus muscle too far cranially, i.e. at the horizontal glabellar line, which does not correspond with the bony origin of the muscle, may also weaken the medial fibers of the frontalis muscle, leading to medial eyebrow ptosis.
- *"Spock" or "Mephisto" shaped eyebrow*
  This complication is a common tell-tale sign of neuromodulator treatment of glabella frown lines. It is caused by lateral hypercontractility of the frontalis muscle, leading to elevation of the tail of the eyebrow. Injecting the procerus muscle too superiorly, at the level of its dermal insertion, can affect the central frontalis muscle, causing both a depression of the medial third of the eyebrow and hypercontractility of the lateral muscle fibers.
- *Upper eyelid ptosis*
  This adverse event is feared after treatment of glabellar frown lines using neuromodulators. If the toxin is injected deeply, rather than superficially at the cutaneous insertion of the corrugator supercilii muscle, the product may migrate through the supraorbital foramen/notch and access the levator palpaebrae superioris muscle intraorbitally, which is responsible for elevation of the upper eyelid.

FOREHEAD REGION

The layered arrangement of the forehead is composed of eight distinct layers:

Layer 1: Skin
Layer 2: Subcutaneous fat (superficial frontal fat compartments)
Layer 3: Suprafrontalis fascia
Layer 4: Frontalis muscle
Layer 5: Retrofrontalis fat
Layer 6: Subfrontalis fascia
Layer 7: Loose areolar tissue (upper forehead), preperiosteal fat (lower lateral forehead)
Layer 8: Periosteum

The frontalis muscle has no bony adhesion. Instead, it is located within a fascial envelope extending from the galea aponeurotica (supra- and subfrontalis fascia) (Ingallina et al. 2022). The suprafrontalis fascia (layer 3) transmits muscle contractions of the frontalis muscle to the overlying skin (layer 1), and the visibility of the muscle contraction is determined by the thickness of the subcutaneous fat layer (layer 2). In some cases, the left and right muscle belly are separated by a central tendon aponeurosis, which leads to an increased muscle fascicle angle with more lateral orientation of the frontalis muscle fascicles (Moqadam et al. 2017). Interestingly, while the lower frontalis muscle acts as an eyebrow elevator (investing into the orbicularis oculi, corrugator supercilii, and procerus muscle), the upper part of the frontalis muscle acts as a hairline depressor. This bidirectional movement converges at a horizontal line (the C-line) at an approximate length of 60% of the total forehead length (Cotofana et al. 2020).

HORIZONTAL FOREHEAD LINES

Forehead lines result from contraction of the frontalis muscle, corresponding to a perpendicular orientation in regard to the muscle contraction pattern. Depending on the muscle's morphology and the presence of an aponeurosis, straight horizontal or wavy lines can be differentiated (Frank et al. 2019). Wavy forehead lines occur when the muscle's fascicle angle increases and fibers are orientated more laterally (Moqadam et al. 2017). Targeting the forehead using neurotoxin injections can reduce transverse horizontal rhytids. The injection technique should depend on the forehead region injected. Deep neuromodulator injection, into the supraperiosteal plane, should be performed cranial to the C-line by needle insertion with slight bone contact (Davidovic et al. 2021). Superficial subdermal injections should be performed below the C-line (Davidovic et al. 2021). Wavy forehead lines can even extend lateral to the temporal crest, requiring injection lateral to the hairline in some cases.

COMMON ADVERSE EVENTS WHEN TREATING THE FOREHEAD REGION

- *Eyebrow ptosis*
  Targeting the lower forehead below the C-line increases the risk of eyebrow ptosis, due to relaxation of the eyebrow elevation fibers of the frontalis muscle. The risk is especially high if injections are performed deeply in this area, rather than subdermally.
- *"Spock" or "Mephisto" shaped eyebrow*
  Lateral eyebrow hyperelevation can result after injecting the central frontalis muscle without lateralization of injection points when injecting horizontal forehead lines.

PAROTIDEO-MASSETERIC REGION

The parotideo-masseteric region greatly defines the shape of the face due to the projection of the masseter muscle. In general, it includes the following layers:

Layer 1: Skin
Layer 2: Subcutaneous fat (middle and lateral cheek fat)
Layer 3: Superficial musculoaponeurotic system (SMAS)
Layer 4: Deep spaces
Layer 5: Parotideo-masseteric fascia

The masseter muscle is found deep to layer 5 (Cotofana and Lachman 2019), together with branches of the facial nerve and the parotid gland (Figure 11.3). It is composed of two muscle bellies with an anterosuperior fiber orientation, which are separated by a strong intramuscular tendon (Lee et al. 2016, 2019). The bony origin of the superficial belly lies at the maxillary process of the zygomatic bone and the inferior border of the zygomatic arch, while the deep belly originates at the deep inferior surface of the zygomatic arch more posteriorly. Both muscle bellies insert at the mandibular angle and the lateral mandible.

Together with the temporalis and pterygoid muscles, the masseter muscle is mainly involved in mastication.

TREATMENT OF MASSETER MUSCLE HYPERTROPHY AND BRUXISM

Neuromodulator treatment of the masseter muscle can reduce masseter muscle volume and strength. Injections can relieve bruxism and/or alter the shape of the face by reducing masseteric projection, thereby leading to facial slimming. In turn, hypertrophy of other muscles of mastication

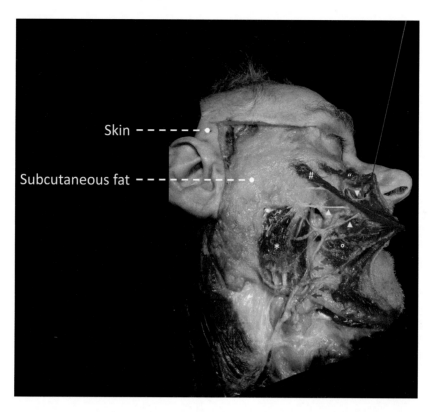

FIGURE 11.3 Cadaveric dissection of the mid- and lower face. The facial vein (blue arrows) and facial artery (red arrows) are exposed in the lower face, at the anterior border of the masseter muscle (*). The masseter muscle is composed of two muscle bellies with an anterosuperior fiber orientation, which are separated by a strong intramuscular tendon. The parotid gland has been removed in this specimen. Branches of the facial nerve are marked as Δ. The buccinator (°) zygomaticus major (#) and levator labii superioris alequae nasi (") muscles are marked. The infraorbital neurovascular bundle is highlighted.

compensating for the relaxation of the masseter muscle may occur. For example, hypertrophy of the temporalis muscle would add additional aesthetic effect in patients with temporal hollowing (Nikolis et al. 2020). Prior to injection, the extension of the masseter muscle should be palpated manually during clenching of the teeth. Care must be taken to inject deep and in bone contact in the lower 25% of the total extent of the muscle in order to penetrate the intramuscular tendon of the masseter muscle, thus targeting the deep head of the muscle.

COMMON ADVERSE EVENTS WHEN TREATING THE PAROTIDEO-MASSETERIC REGION

- *Asymmetrical smile*
  Too superficial administration of the neurotoxin, i.e. targeting only the superficial head of the masseter muscle without penetration of the intramuscular tendon, might lead to retrograde migration of the product and relaxation of the superficial risorius muscle, thereby causing an asymmetrical smile.
- *Masseter bulging*
  Injections of the deep masseter belly only can cause paradoxical bulging of the superficial belly, as the neurotoxin might be restricted to the deep belly by the deep inferior tendon. Both compartments should be injected for optimal results.

LOWER FACE, JAWLINE, AND CHIN

The contour of the jawline is of great importance for facial attractiveness. It has a classic five-layered arrangement:

Layer 1: Skin
Layer 2: Subcutaneous fat (i.e. jowl fat compartment)
Layer 3: Platysma and depressor anguli oris muscle
Layer 4: Subplatysmal fat and deep fat
Layer 5: Periosteum

The platysma muscle majorly determines the tone and positioning of the jawline. It is the main facial depressor muscle, as it ascends over the anterolateral aspect of the neck in a superomedial trajectory, connecting to the superior aspect of the depressor labii inferioris, to the modiolus and extending past the mandibular angle (Figure 11.4). It is continuous with the SMAS and the orbicularis oculi muscle in the midface and the superficial temporal fascia in the upper face (Cotofana et al. 2016) (Figure 11.5). The platysma muscle is highly mobile, as it has no direct connection to the underlying mandible. The inferior displacement of the midfacial fat compartments as well as gravitational effects during aging contribute to a caudal displacement of the platysma muscle and the overlying jowl fat compartment, thereby leading to jowl deformity (Suwanchinda et al. 2018).

The shape of the chin corresponds mainly to the underlying mentalis muscle (Figure 11.6). It has its bony origin inferior to the labiomental sulcus. The muscle fibers travel inferiorly and insert

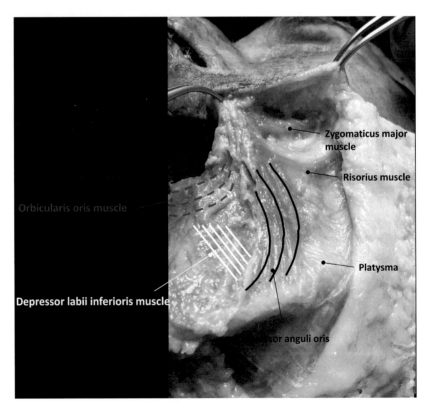

FIGURE 11.4   Cadaveric dissection of the lower face after removal of the skin and subcutaneous fat, depicting the perioral region and the perioral musculature, including the depressor labii inferioris muscle, depressor anguli oris muscle, orbicularis oris muscle, platysma, risorius, and zygomaticus major muscle.

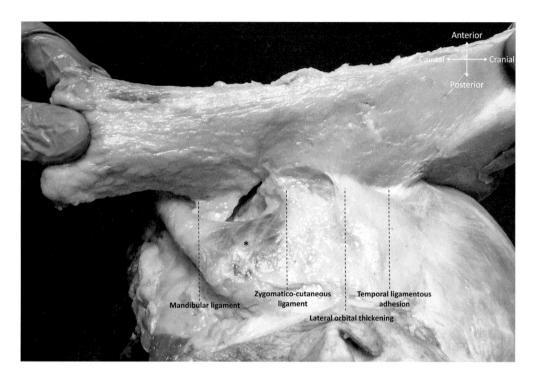

FIGURE 11.5 Cadaveric dissection of the left hemiface showing the continuous layered arrangement of the face. The subcutaneous fat and superficial musculo-aponeurotic system (including superficial temporal fascia, SMAS, and the platysma) are elevated together. Note the facial ligaments. The masseter muscle (*) is covered by the parotideomasseteric fascia.

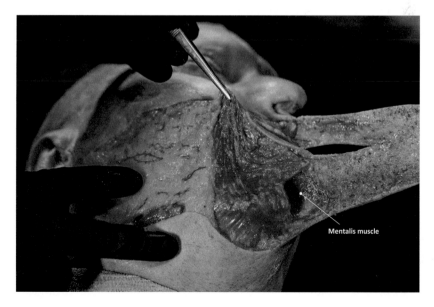

FIGURE 11.6 Cadaveric dissection of the lower face depicting the bony origin of the mentalis muscle, which inserts superficially into the subcutaneous fat and dermis.

directly into the dermis. Mentalis muscle contraction elevates the chin and everts the lower lip. Dimpling of the overlying skin can occur due to the dermal fiber insertions.

JAWLINE CONTOURING USING NEUROTOXIN

Injection of neurotoxin into the platysma muscle can alleviate tension of the muscle, thus antagonizing its inferior pull and aligning the contour of the underlying mandible. Additionally, mild elevation of the lateral face can be perceived, as the lateral face depressor is paralyzed. This can increase midfacial volume and reduce jowl deformity. Multiple injection points should be administered subdermally, approximately 1 cm cranial to the mandibular line. Medially injections should extend to 1 cm inferior of the oral commissure (Swift et al. 2022). Moreover, platysmal bands should be targeted, further impacting the aesthetic outcome for the patient.

TREATMENT OF THE CHIN

Neuromodulator treatment of the chin can have multiple effects. Deep injections in the midline with bone contact weaken the activity of the mentalis muscle, smoothen the labiomandibular sulcus, and feminize facial appearance by elongating the chin and by changing it from square to heart shaped. Furthermore, superficial subdermal injections can reduce skin surface dimpling.

COMMON ADVERSE EVENTS WHEN TREATING THE LOWER FACE

- *Lower lip asymmetry*
  Deep injection of neurotoxin medial to the labiomandibular sulcus can paralyze the depressor labii inferioris muscle. Imprecise product administration both for platysma or mentalis injections can thus result in asymmetric lip movement and disturbance of oral commissure closure.

EFFECTS OF NEUROTOXIN INJECTIONS ON THE SKIN

The skin covers the entire external surface of the human body and is considered the largest human organ. It provides a protective physical barrier against mechanical stress, pathogens, ultraviolet light, and toxins. Its major functions include temperature regulation, immune defense, transportation of sensory information, and homeostasis (Lopez-Ojeda et al. 2021). In the face, it varies with regard to thickness, adhesion to underlying fascial layers, pigmentation, and coloration, depending on the facial region. While the skin is comparably thick in the midface, it is thin and transparent in the infraorbital region and has direct attachments to the underlying orbicularis oculi muscle. The lack of a subcutaneous fat layer in this region accounts for the bluish pigmentation of the area, reflecting the color of the muscle fibers (Cotofana et al. 2015). Medial to the nasolabial and labiomandibular sulcus, the skin has strong attachments to an interwoven collagen–muscle fiber meshwork with subcutaneous fat being interposed between this network, connecting the skin with the muscles of facial expression.

The effects of neurotoxin injections on the skin itself are discussed controversially. Frequent and long-term injection of neurotoxin could cause atrophy of terminal muscle fibers within the dermis and the three-dimensional SMAS network, leading to thinning of the skin. On the other hand, studies have suggested that an increase in elasticity and pliability of the treated skin occurs (Bonaparte & Ellis 2015). These controversies highlight the need for further high-quality research in this regard.

BODY CONTOURING USING NEUROTOXIN INJECTIONS

Apart from the treatment of facial rhytids, neuromodulators can be utilized for several different indications, including body sculpting procedures. The aim is to cause muscular atrophy, rather than relaxation, as is the case when treating the face. Similar to the treatment of muscle spasticity, high doses of neurotoxin are injected deep into the muscular tissue, causing slimming and definition of the treated area. Common examples include injections into the trapezius, biceps, triceps, deltoid, or gastrocnemius muscles (Yi et al. 2020; Cheng et al. 2020).

CLOSING REMARKS

Much of what happens at the skin surface can be extrapolated to the underlying musculature. Patients often consult practitioners of aesthetic medicine to ameliorate facial rhytids, which can be achieved by muscle paralysis using neurotoxins. Importantly, facial muscles do not act individually but are interwoven in muscle complexes composed of agonists and antagonists, enabling most complex facial expressions. Here, the paralysis of a single muscle causes a disequilibrium which needs to be taken into account and anticipated by the injector. The treating physician must foresee all consequences following the aesthetic treatment and aim for the most accurate and predictable injections, especially when injecting neurotoxins. Profound knowledge of the underlying anatomy and individualized assessment will guide injectors toward safer, more efficient, and more precise results, with less collateral damage.

REFERENCES

Ahsanuddin S, Roy S, Nasser W, Povolotskiy R, Paskhover B. Adverse events associated with Botox as reported in a food and drug administration database. *Aesthetic Plast Surg.* 2021;45(3):1201–1209.

Bonaparte JP, Ellis D. Alterations in the elasticity, pliability, and viscoelastic properties of facial skin after injection of Onabotulinum Toxin A. *JAMA Facial Plast Surg.* 2015;17(4):256–263.

Cheng J, Chung HJ, Friedland M, Hsu SH. Botulinum toxin injections for leg contouring in East Asians. *Dermatol Surg.* 2020;46(Suppl 1):S62–S70.

Cotofana S, Schenck TL, Trevidic P, et al. Midface: Clinical anatomy and regional approaches with injectable fillers. *Plast Reconstr Surg.* 2015;136(5 Suppl):219S–234S.

Cotofana S, Fratila AA, Schenck TL, Redka-Swoboda W, Zilinsky I, Pavicic T. The anatomy of the aging face: A review. *Facial Plast Surg.* 2016;32(3):253–260.

Cotofana S, Freytag DL, Frank K, et al. The bidirectional movement of the frontalis muscle: Introducing the line of convergence and its potential clinical relevance. *Plast Reconstr Surg.* 2020;145(5):1155–1162.

Cotofana S, Lachman N. Anatomy of the facial fat compartments and their relevance in aesthetic surgery. *J Dtsch Dermatol Ges.* 2019;17(4):399–413.

Cotofana S, Pedraza AP, Kaufman J, et al. Respecting upper facial anatomy for treating the glabella with neuromodulators to avoid medial brow ptosis – A refined 3-point injection technique. *J Cosmet Dermatol.* 2021;20(6):1625–1633.

Davidovic K, Melnikov DV, Frank K, et al. To click or not to click – The importance of understanding the layers of the forehead when injecting neuromodulators – A clinical, prospective, interventional, split-face study. *J Cosmet Dermatol.* 2021;20(5):1385–1392.

Frank K, Freytag DL, Schenck TL, et al. Relationship between forehead motion and the shape of forehead lines-A 3D skin displacement vector analysis. *J Cosmet Dermatol.* 2019. PMID: 31282119.

Ingallina F, Frank K, Mardini S, et al. Re-evaluation of the layered anatomy of the forehead – introducing the subfrontalis fascia and the retro-frontalis fat compartments. *Plast Reconstr Surg* 2022. PMID: 35006205.

Lee HJ, Choi YJ, Lee KW, Hu KS, Kim ST, Kim HJ. Ultrasonography of the internal architecture of the superficial part of the masseter muscle in vivo. *Clin Anat.* 2019;32(3):446–452.

Lee HJ, Kang IW, Seo KK, et al. The anatomical basis of Paradoxical masseteric bulging after botulinum neurotoxin type A injection. *Toxins (Basel)* 2016;9(1).

Lopez-Ojeda W, Pandey A, Alhajj M, Oakley AM. Anatomy, Skin (Integument). In: StatPearls. Treasure Island (FL), 2021.

Moqadam M, Frank K, Handayan C, et al. Understanding the shape of forehead lines. *J Drugs Dermatol.* 2017;16(5):471–477.

Nikolis A, Enright KM, Rudolph C, Cotofana S. Temporal volume increase after reduction of masseteric hypertrophy utilizing incobotulinumtoxin type A. *J Cosmet Dermatol.* 2020;19(6):1294–1300.

Sandulescu T, Buechner H, Rauscher D, Naumova EA, Arnold WH. Histological, SEM and three-dimensional analysis of the midfacial SMAS – New morphological insights. *Ann Anat.* 2019;222:70–78.

Small R. Botulinum toxin injection for facial wrinkles. *American Family Physician.* 2014;90(3):168–175.

Suwanchinda A, Rudolph C, Hladik C, et al. The layered anatomy of the jawline. *J Cosmet Dermatol.* 2018;17(4):625–631.

Swift A, Green JB, Hernandez CA, et al. Tips and tricks for facial toxin injections with illustrated anatomy. *Plast Reconstr Surg.* 2022;149(2):303e–312e.

Sykes JM, Cotofana S, Trevidic P, et al. Upper face: Clinical anatomy and regional approaches with injectable fillers. *Plast Reconstr Surg.* 2015;136(5 Suppl):204S–218S.

Yi KH, Lee HJ, Choi YJ, Lee K, Lee JH, Kim HJ. Anatomical guide for botulinum neurotoxin injection: Application to cosmetic shoulder contouring, pain syndromes, and cervical dystonia. *Clin Anat.* 2020. doi.org/10.1002/ca.23690

12 Why Injection Depth Is Important for Better Aesthetic Toxin Practice

Yates Yen-Yu Chao

CONTENTS

The usual guidance on toxin injection specifies the number of units and the points of injection based on surface landmarks but is less concerned with injection depth. However, toxin that works on the neuromuscular junction has to be delivered as close as possible to the target endplate or inside the muscle. A precise toxin practice should be done with the right dosage, fit the muscle distribution, and be appropriate in depth. However, surface landmarks correlate only loosely with the underlying structures. The depth of injection should adapt to regional tissue layering relationships and tissue thickness. Locating the points of injection should not be based solely on the distance to certain surface points.

MUSCLE THICKNESS AND SKIN THICKNESS

As toxin is ideally to be delivered directly to the muscle to reach the endplate structure as soon as possible, the distance to the muscle at a certain point from the overlying surface skin should be the intended depth of injection. The thickness of skin and amount of adipose tissue in between could vary with gender, age, ethnic traits, BMI (body mass index), personal features, and the exact location of injection. Ultrasound images can facilitate the determination of tissue thickness but increase the awkwardness of a quick procedure.

It is equally important to administer toxin at an adequate depth to decrease the necessity of the toxin having to spread to achieve its effect and to limit unnecessarily deep penetration of the needle to avoid unwanted toxin effects (Figure 12.1). This is more important when different muscles are stratified in a limited space. That means the placement of the needle tip is critical with respect to the thickness and layering of tissue to avoid complications arising from toxin injection. Muscle thickness can be an issue of concern in the opposite way, in that a bulky muscle might need more than a single shot to cover all the muscle fibers across the muscle span (Figure 12.2a,b and 12.3a,b). Some of the fibers that have not been deadened show twitching after treatment on a bulky muscle if the injection targeted only the superficial or the deep part.

Information about the thickness of skin and muscle should be gathered before injection by anatomical knowledge and assessment by visual means, palpation, and exercise.

DOI: 10.1201/9781003008132-12

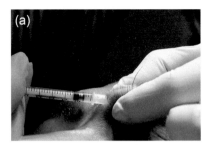 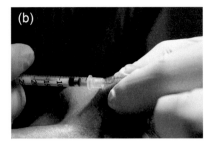

FIGURE 12.1 A corrugator toxin injection is ideally conducted as an intramuscular injection. (a) The injection needle can reach deeper on the medial side as the origin of the corrugator is the deepest part of the muscle, which starts at the orbital rim. (b) The lateral tail of the corrugator can be approached more superficially as it inserts into the supraorbital skin.

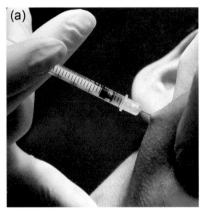 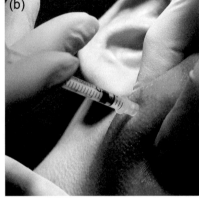

FIGURE 12.2 The masseter muscle is a bulky muscle with multiple compartments. (a) The usual insulin syringes with a fixed short needle can hardly reach the deep compartment; (b) they should be employed only for superficial doses.

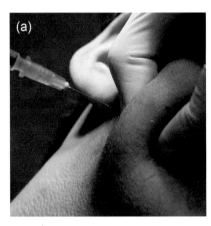 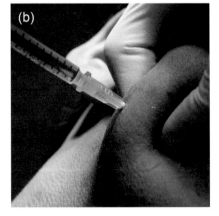

FIGURE 12.3 (a,b) To have a complete effect for the lower masseter, syringes with detachable needles are long enough to reach the deeper compartment of masseter muscles.

DEPTH CONCERNS FOR COMMON FACIAL INDICATIONS

The common indications of facial aesthetic treatment represent three different patterns of the skin-to-muscle relationship that can be the models for toxin injection study.

- *Crow's feet*

  The target for crow's feet treatment is the lateral arcade of the orbicularis oculi muscle. The orbicularis oculi is a very thin layer of muscle with its myofibers distributed immediately below the skin, with barely a trace of intervening adipose tissue. The periorbital skin which covers the thin layer of muscle is the thinnest in the human body. Compared with the other areas of the face, the upper eyelid has skin about 0.4 mm thick, including epidermis and dermis, which is less than one-third of the skin thickness on the nasal tip. Injection of toxins in this area must be superficial enough. The level of needle penetration when the needle is inserted vertically into the skin is about the immersion of the bevel. Oblique insertion with the tip pointed to the lateral is usually described for a crow's feet injection. However, a vertical insertion with strictly controlled depth of needle penetration is more precise, eliminating the variable of needle direction on both sides (Figure 12.4). The bevel should be kept with the opening upwards. Compared with the entire extent of orbicularis oculi, the extent of the toxin block is small. The requirement for toxin spread is limited. The injection volume should be minimized per aliquot, or toxin should be reconstituted more densely to help to facilitate treatment precision. Deep injection of toxin at the lateral canthal margin might result in unwanted side effects on the function of the levator muscles of the zygomaticus. Deep injection in this area is not recommended because zygomaticus muscles are deeply stratified, and the desired toxin effect on the orbicularis oculi will need toxin diffusion back from a deep injection.

- *Frown lines*

  The corrugator is the main muscle that needs to be blocked in order to reduce the glabella frown line. This muscle has an attachment to the orbital rim at the medial superior corner and upper tethering fibers connecting to the superficial skin at the lateral end, about the middle of the eyebrow. The muscle extends from deep bone to the superficial across several tissue layers and varies in depth throughout. The oblique insertion pattern causes

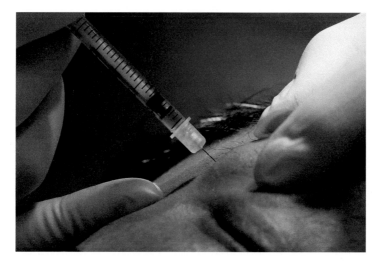

FIGURE 12.4   The author prefers vertical injection for the lateral canthal skin to make sure the delivery of toxin is symmetrical for crow's feet on both sides.

only limited problems in terms of judging injection depth because the bony attachment is not very deep in structure and the muscle is small and short. The entire muscle is about 38–53 mm long and 1 cm wide at its lateral origin. The most medial insertion part of the muscle is about 5.7 mm in depth and the most lateral part 6.6 mm in depth. The corrugator muscle span is visually detectable by the resulting wrinkle and dimpling at the superficial insertion point. The muscle belly is palpable and can be pinched with the fingers. Precise delivery of botulinum toxin can be achieved by direct muscle insertion. Complete coverage of the small muscle can be accomplished by one or two shots of toxin without too much toxin spread. As the muscle runs up approaching lateral, the injecting needle should be inserted more deeply in the medial head and more superficially if the lateral end is intended (Figure 12.1a,b). Ideally, the toxin indicated here should be thicker to avoid spread to the nearby extraocular muscles or levator aponeurosis, especially when injecting high doses of toxin for strengthful corrugators.

The injection pattern for this is obviously different from that for crow's feet; intradermal or superficial injection is not preferred as the muscle stays a little deeper. Superficial injection here would need to work via diffusion, being less efficient and precise. Injecting doses are higher as the muscle fibers are grouped together as a belly. The number of toxin doses per shot should be dependent on the volume of muscle, but techniques are similar in their relative delicacy and the existence of nearby muscles that need precision in toxin distribution.

- *Forehead*

  The frontalis muscle presents as a thin layer of broad muscle covering almost the whole forehead area, connecting with the galea, and interdigitating about the brow ridge with the skin. The whole extent of the muscle stays close above the frontal cranium, below the forehead skin and adipose tissue. In contrast to the orbicularis oculi muscle, it is much larger and broader and situated a little deeper. The forehead skin could be much thicker than the periorbital skin. All these factors necessitate the adjustment of the toxin injection for better efficacy and thorough coverage.

  However, the traditional guideline for the forehead injection does not look that different from that for crow's feet, either in the number of units per shot or the number of injection points when counting both sides of lateral canthus together. A simple survey of the instruction for forehead injection on the internet and in the literature can easily reveal the obviously similar regimes for dosing and reconstitution for the two muscles that looks conflicting. If limited shots of toxin can succeed on the forehead, the toxin must have worked through considerable toxin spread (Figure 12.5a,b). However, that kind of spreading tendency could be dangerous and harmful for the lateral canthal injections.

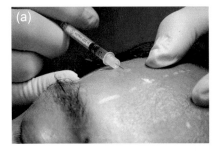 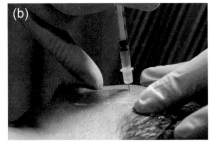

FIGURE 12.5 The practice of forehead injection is variable. (a) A superficial injection of toxin has to deliver the toxin to the muscle structure through deep diffusion. (b) A vertical supraperiosteal injection delivers the toxin more closely to the muscle, but toxin has to diffuse back to have an inhibiting function on the sweat glands. This variable is more prominent in patients with thick skin and more adipose tissue. That is one of the reasons different diffusion studies reach different conclusions, even when the injection depth is kept constant at a certain number of millimeters.

THE CHALLENGES OF EFFECTIVE TOXIN DELIVERY BY APPROPRIATE INJECTION DEPTH

From the author's experiences teaching aesthetic toxin treatments, injectors seem encountering more problems treating forehead lines as compared to the treatment for lateral canthal folds or frown lines. The reasons for suboptimal toxin effects for forehead lines include concomitant ptosis in some patients with pre-existing periorbital tissue laxity and the broadness of the frontalis muscle, which presents a challenge to achieving a homogeneous and adequate coverage of the entire area.

Many instructions for forehead toxin injection involve only 4–6 points of injection. If limited shots can calm down this broad piece of muscle, then toxin spread must play an important role in the whole process. Toxin spread is an issue occurring in both horizontal and vertical directions. The depth of toxin injection on the forehead matters considering the layered frontal structure, however, injection depth was less addressed in the treatment of forehead lines. A simple survey of videos on the internet could easily find many of the practices injecting toxin on the forehead dispense toxin very superficially, not too differently from the injection of the lateral orbit. When toxin is injected superficially, like intradermal injection the toxin molecule has to spread across the dermis, adipose soft tissue, and fascia to reach the muscle to ensure the inhibition effect. Toxin injection in the wrong layer could waste the product, decrease treatment efficacy, and create more residual muscle contraction, especially when the toxin reconstitution is more concentrated or the toxin product is featured with less spreading tendency.

TREATING MUSCLES BY DIFFUSION

When forehead toxin treatment is undergone with limited injection points and high dose injection, spreading plays an important role in completing the clinical effects. However, any treatment that relies on toxin spreading is risky and imprecise.

Usually, limited spots of injection are coupled with larger units per injection as the limited points of inhibition effect need a larger working diameter to cover the muscle adequately. Though toxin injection in this way has been done for a period of time and could suffice for coverage, the arrangement of toxin points and doses could be refined further to be more precise in effect and meet more delicate or individualized needs. It is easy to see that the safe zone of toxin injection had been set higher to avoid unwanted drooping eyebrows or eyelid heaviness. As we know for the diffusion pattern of large unit injection and diluted toxin injection, to cover a certain area with large circles of diffusion toxin, there must be overlapping areas that resulted in waste. For delicate structures and crowded muscles diffusion would result in imprecision (large circle to fit in small rooms). Large unit injection usually has the center of injection as an overdosed area and a wider spreading diameter with decreasing concentration gradient. That is why these practices use more toxin than new injection methods, while the extent of muscle inhibition does not differ that much.

When examining the diffusion issue for a broad muscle, another thing we have to keep in mind is the appropriateness of traditional reconstitution recommendations. It is interesting that the same formula for toxin reconstitution is used for both frontal broadness and the corrugator or orbicularis oculi muscles. Considering the big difference in muscle size, if similar number of injection points and the similar dose per injection are right for the forehead, it could be dangerous for the lateral canthal area. If it is appropriate for crow's feet, then the coverage for the forehead could be incomplete.

The author usually prepares toxin in two different concentrations. For small muscles (like levator labii superioris alaeque nasi) or indications that need restricted distribution (like mouth angle elevation), toxin with less reconstituting saline can give more precise effects. For big muscles (like the soleus) and indications that require spreading (like the forehead), toxin of the standard reconstituting concentration can be employed with reasonable spread. The toxin concentration and injection method can be modified accordingly to better suit different structural and functional requirements (see Chapter 16).

BIBLIOGRAPHY

Choi YJ, et al. Ultrasonographic analyses of the forehead region for injectable treatments. *Ultrasound Med Biol* 2019;45(10):2641–2648.

Davidovic K, et al. To click or not to click – The importance of understanding the layers of the forehead when injecting neuromodulators – A clinical, prospective, interventional, split-face study. *J Cosmet Dermatol* 2021;20(5):1385–1392.

Ha RY, et al. Analysis of facial skin thickness: Defining the relative thickness index. *Plast Reconstr Surg* 2005;115(6):1769–1773.

Kaplan JB, et al. Consideration of muscle depth for botulinum toxin injections: A three-dimensional approach. *Plast Surg Nurs* 2019;39(2):52–58.

Kim YS, et al. Regional thickness of facial skin and superficial fat: Application to the minimally invasive procedures. *Clin Anat* 2019;32(8):1008–1018.

Lee KW, et al. Validity and reliability of a structured-light 3D scanner and an ultrasound imaging system for measurements of facial skin thickness. *Clin Anat* 2017;30(7):878–886.

Pellacani G, et al. Variations in facial skin thickness and echogenicity with site and age. *Acta Derm Venereol* 1999;79(5):366–369.

Trévidic P, et al. Anatomy of the lower face and botulinum toxin injections. *Plast Reconstr Surg* 2015;136(5 Suppl):84S–91S.

13 Distributing Toxin Precisely to the Motor Endplates

Yates Yen-Yu Chao

CONTENTS

Most commercial kits of botulinum toxin A contain serotype A units, which exert their pharmaceutical effect through a multistep process at the neuromuscular junction. Injection of the toxin as close to the nerve terminal as possible is important to facilitate the precision and efficiency of toxin peptides uptake and reduce toxin waste, attain a quicker onset of clinical reaction, and avoid aberrant spread and unnecessary inhibition of neighboring muscles.

The traditional understanding of the nerve-to-muscle interface in the extrafusal muscle fibers of human skeletal muscles is a center-located narrow band of motor endplates (MEP) (Figure 13.1). However, the exact architecture of different muscles and the innervation pattern are much more complex than the assumption of muscle center distribution. In aesthetic practice, botulinum toxin is rarely targeted merely at the center. The forehead myofibers of the frontalis muscle extend from the hairline to the eyebrow, interdigitating with orbicularis oculi muscle. If the MEPs of the frontalis muscle are all distributed about the midline of the muscle as a band, the effect of toxin should vary in intensity according to how many light chains reach that band. However, that seems to conflict with our experience, as we split our dosages into different shots; toxin injection of the forehead is generally reserved for the upper portion to avoid worsening the problem of eyelid or brow ptosis. Forehead toxin injection has even been designed in a V-shaped distribution to augment the pattern of the eyebrow arch. Muscle structures and the MEP distribution should be different from and more complex than what is taught in traditional myology (Figure 13.2).

There have been anatomical articles describing muscle innervation and toxin injection points based on the observation of nerve arborization. It has been suggested that toxin be administered near the nerve bundle to enhance treatment efficiency. However, aesthetic toxin practice should be driven by aesthetic purposes to achieve a better morphological presentation rather than to paralyze a muscle as completely as possible. A judgment should be made so that our dosing and spatial allocations of toxin injection are adjusted to follow the right parameters.

MUSCLE ARCHITECTURE AND THE DISTRIBUTION OF MEPs

The physical arrangement of muscle fibers plays a decisive role in a muscle's mechanical function. Body muscles where toxin has been used for aesthetic moderation have different arrangements: fan-shaped parallel fibers in the trapezius muscle, fusiform parallel fibers in the biceps brachii,

DOI: 10.1201/9781003008132-13

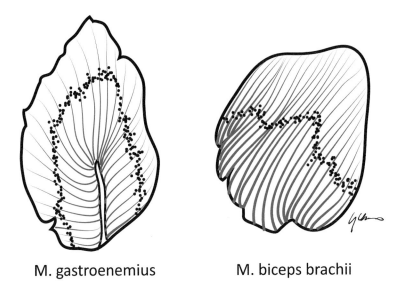

M. gastroenemius   M. biceps brachii

FIGURE 13.1   Traditional understanding of the distribution of MEPs. (Adapted from Pospisilova and Parizek 1976.)

bipennate fibers and unipennate fibers in the triceps and gastrocnemius, and multipennate fibers in the soleus and deltoid muscles. According to earlier studies using a special stain, most endplates are distributed in the middle of muscle fibers, while endplates aggregate as convex or more complex curving bands in pennate muscles.

Facial muscle studies using similar methods reveal more variable patterns of MEP distribution. One-quarter of the facial muscles have multiple MEPs on one muscle fiber. All facial muscles are flat in shape, except the orbicularis oris muscle. The zygomatic minor muscle is the only one that is rectangular in shape, while the depressor labii inferioris is quadrilateral-shaped, and all other muscles are trapezoid in shape, converging from a wider origin to a narrow insertion (Figure 13.3). Differently from body muscle, MEPs are always located in an eccentric position and never in the middle of the fiber bundle. When a muscle is innervated by different nerve branches, MEPs are clustered as several motor zones near the nerve entrance points. However, the orbicularis oculi and oris muscles are devoid of band-like motor zones but have the disseminated MEPs evenly distributed on the entire muscle sheet. Unlike body muscles, a great number of fibers were identified as having more than one MEP. Polyneuronal innervation was suggested for the complex expressional and emotional muscle excursion.

As the histological and electrophysiological evidence about mammalian and human muscles grows, the traditional understanding of MEP and neuromuscular interaction has been revised to show that one muscle fiber can contain multiple endplates and MEPs can be located eccentrically or evenly distributed throughout the muscle.

POINTS OF INJECTION MATTER

Often in the training for botulinum toxin injection, injection points and injection units are taught according to anatomical muscle distribution and wrinkle patterns. However, these points may not be related to the exact points of MEP distribution.

Botulinum toxins start their effect by binding to the nerve terminals and internalization of the functional peptide. The binding of toxins to the nerve-cell membrane involves a series of protein–lipid and protein–protein interactions with cellular membrane components. The ganglioside that

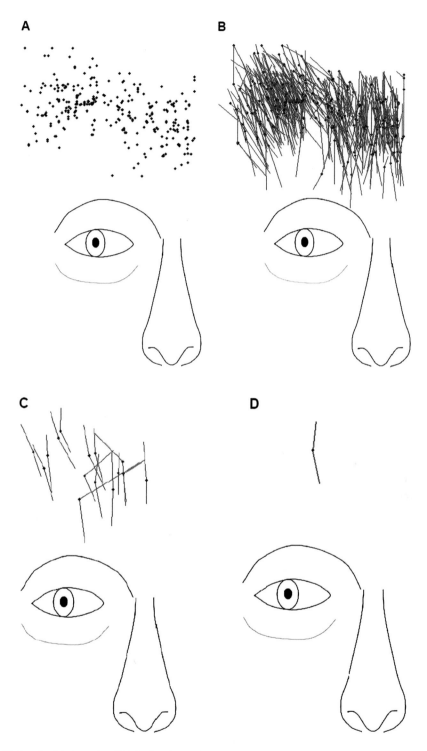

FIGURE 13.2 (A–D) A study of high-density surface electromyography measured the facial muscles about the distribution of motor endplates. MEPs are predominantly localized in the upper forehead and are spread evenly throughout the area, and can be divided into a medial and a lateral cluster. The superior fibers are oriented in a cranial and craniolateral direction; the inferior fibers were in a caudal and caudomedial direction. (From Neubert 2016.)

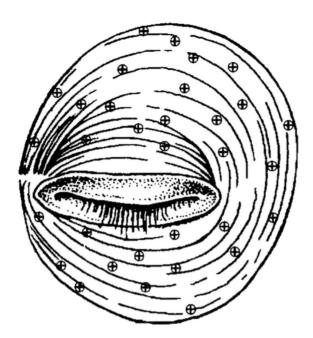

FIGURE 13.3 A study on human cadavers staining the MEPs found that there is no specific "motor zone" in some muscles. For example, in the orbicularis oculi muscle, the MEPs are evenly spread over the muscle. (From Happak et al. 1997, with permission.)

mediates toxin internalization is highly concentrated at presynaptic terminals, and the synaptic structures are known as the MEP where the nerve endings meet the muscle. In a large or broad muscle, botulinum toxin should be preferably administered near the target of MEPs to achieve better efficacy. In one study, the MEP area of the extensor digitorum brevis was localized using high-density surface EMG to validate the clinical efficacy of endplate targeting injection. Toxin injected at a distance of 12 mm away from the MEP area has to be double in dosage compared with direct onsite delivery.

Botulinum toxin used for aesthetic purposes is ideally kept in as low a dose as possible to avoid spread to neighboring muscle, exerting unnecessary block.

FOLLOW THE NERVE OR FOLLOW THE MUSCLE?

With the advances in the practice of aesthetic toxin injection, the importance of anatomical knowledge has been well recognized. Most teachings about toxin injection include anatomical information about the target muscles and their innervation. Identifying the shape and location of the target muscle is the first step, wherein the toxin is to be injected into the invisible muscle underlying the surface skin through which needles are being inserted. It is easily understandable that the distribution and shape of a muscle that we intend to decrease in function should be related to the points of injection. However, the MEPs are not evenly spread throughout the muscles.

Nerve branching and histological evidence of muscular innervation pattern have been used as maps to guide toxin injection to achieve better toxin efficacy. However, the toxin works through the presynaptic nerve membrane, not the nerve trunk or branch itself. Branch density follows the en plaque area (the en plaque area full of motor endplates has denser distribution of nerve endings), but the very fine terminals extend further.

The judgment for a correct deployment of botulinum toxin is crucial to achieve a precise and better aesthetic result and to reduce toxin waste and unwanted side effects. Morphological information on the muscle underlying the skin is the most fundamental parameter for the practitioner to administer toxin within the right territory, reducing erroneous denervation of neighboring muscles.

But the arrangement of toxin shots within a muscle and the split of toxin dose across the muscle span should take the distribution of MEPs into consideration as well.

Instead of treating a muscle with widespread toxin, it would be preferable not to bombard the MEP area if it is localized as the switch of the muscle. Aesthetic treatment through muscle moderation should do anything but paralyze a certain unit. The success of a toxin treatment should not be determined by the efficiency of its inhibition but by the achievement of a desirable facial appearance or dynamicity. Careful doctors usually allocate injection points as a design to selectively block part of the muscle, altering facial landmark position and facial or body contours, and calming down some muscular overactivity. However, this selective dosing or wrinkle elimination is not always coherent as the MEP distribution limits the toxin's functioning to an intended area and pattern. Usually, a peripheral nerve trunk has several branches. When the nerve reaches the muscle, it sends out several in-muscle branches. Each of the branches corresponds to one MEP lamella cluster. Submaximal contractions are usually the recruitment of a number of the motor units from different lamella clusters. A muscle can be divided into several subgroups of muscle fibers. Toxin molecules that have been placed selectively when reaching the MEPs of the fibers in that range would mean that the toxin would have its effect not far from the plot of injection sites. But the doses near the MEP bands or center would certainly have a more direct effect than those for the eccentric spots.

INJECTION STRATEGY FOR COMMON INDICATIONS

Aesthetic toxin treatments should always be careful, delicate, and done with the utmost craftsmanship. Premium techniques of toxin moderation should be individualized and selective.

FOREHEAD

The endplates of the frontalis muscle are predominantly localized in the upper half up and down in a band-shaped area. In one-third of subjects, these endplates are clustered into medial and lateral groups. The lateral fibers and vector are tilted to the lateral while the medial ones are more vertical. Endplate distribution reaches lower when approaching the medial group. The traditional forehead injection covers some of these hot zones. Partial inhibition of the frontalis fiber raises the brow arch and pulls it laterally. Selective injections in fibers away from the lower portion of the forehead maintain the function of the lower motor units and a basic tone, keeping the brow position (see Chapter 16); these inferior fibers should have their MEPs out of the hot zones that keep them not to be affected by the superior injections.

CROW'S FEET

Endplates are uniquely widespread throughout the orbicularis oculi muscle. Motor units in different regions of the muscle comply with the fiber orientation and distribution, providing vectors in different directions. The disseminated distribution of MEPs within the muscle allows a more careful arrangement of injections to modify muscle activity, decreasing wrinkle extent and the magnitude of the opposing forces interacting with the frontalis (Figure 13.4a,b).

MASSETER

The endplate zone of the masseter is more active in the lower part, 40–50mm from the zygomatic arch. The MEPs of the masseter are not centered but are spread over the muscle fibers. The usual practice of toxin injection on the masseter is restricted by its selective inhibition and focal effect to avoid loss of function of the entire masseter (see Chapter 18).

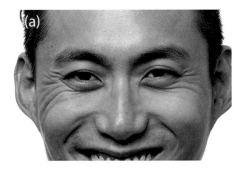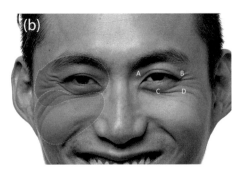

FIGURE 13.4 Lateral canthal lines are the result of muscle contraction in the lateral orbit. (a) The folding of skin extends further laterally and inferiorly, merging with the wrinkles and contributing to the contraction of zygomaticus major and minor. Disseminated distribution of MEP in orbicularis oculi allows the careful design of toxin injection around the eye to have more desirable results. (b) However, the placement of toxin should be conservative in these exaggerated wrinkles, rather than attacking every line. Complete immobilization should be avoided to maintain harmony with other highly mobile areas.

BIBLIOGRAPHY

Akaaboune M, et al. Rapid and reversible effects of activity on acetylcholine receptor density at the neuromuscular junction in vivo. *Science* 1999; 286:503–507.

Arribas M, et al. High resolution labeling of cholinergic nerve terminals using a specific fully active biotinylated botulinum neurotoxin type A. *J Neurosci Res* 1993;36(6):635–645.

Elwischger K, et al. Intramuscular distribution of botulinum toxin – visualized by MRI. *J Neurol Sci* 2014;344(1–2):76–79.

Ezure H. Development of the motor endplates in the masseter muscle in the human fetus. *Ann Anat* 1996;178(1):15–23.

Fawcett PR, et al. Comparison of electrophysiological and histochemical methods for assessing the spatial distribution of muscle fibres of a motor unit within muscle. *J Neurol Sci* 1985;69(1–2):67–79.

Gans C, et al. Muscle architecture in relation to function. *J Biomech* 1991;24(Suppl 1):53–65.

Happak W, et al. Human facial muscles: Dimensions, motor endplate distribution, and presence of muscle fibers with multiple motor endplates. *Anat Rec* 1997;249(2):276–840.

Iwasaki S, et al. Noninvasive estimation of the location of the end plate in the human masseter muscle using surface electromyograms with an electrode array. *J Osaka Dent Univ* 1990;24(2):135–140.

Lapatki BG, et al. Topographical characteristics of motor units of the lower facial musculature revealed by means of high-density surface EMG. *J Neurophysiol* 2006;95:342–354.

McGill KC. Surface electromyogram signal modelling. *Med Biol Eng Comput* 2004;42(4):446–454.

Neubert, J. Topographical characterization of the upper facial musculature revealed by means of high-density surface electromyography. Open Access Repositorium der Universität Ulm und Technischen Hochschule Ulm. Dissertation, 2016; doi:10.18725/OPARU-4075

Pospisilova B, Parizek J. Comparative study of distribution of motor-end-plates in the muscles of the hind limb of some laboratory animals and the lower limb of man. *Suppl. Sbor. ved. praci Hradec Kralove* 1976; 19:411–422.

Rogozhin AA, et al. Recovery of mouse neuromuscular junctions from single and repeated injections of botulinum neurotoxin A. *J Physiol* 2008;586(13):3163–82.

Yin X, et al. Spatial distribution of motor endplates and its adaptive change in skeletal muscle. *Theranostics* 2019;9(3):734–746.

14 Individualized Aesthetic Toxin Practice or Freestyle Injection?

Yates Yen-Yu Chao

CONTENTS

With the evolution of botulinum toxin application for aesthetic purposes, the techniques and principles of toxin injection are becoming more and more diversified. Even with so many classification systems differentiating wrinkle patterns and muscle dynamicity, they cannot be complete enough to cover all these subtle variations of wrinkle patterns and the background anatomical factors. As more and more knowledge of the underlying mechanism of muscle actions and toxin functions is gained, traditional protocols of toxin injection appear relatively elementary and incomplete, covering problems of divergent origins. However, with the rising of numerous injection skills, novel ideas should also be examined carefully for their scientific reasons, long-term safety, and reproducibility.

THE CLASSIC REVIEW

FOREHEAD LINES

Treatment of horizontal forehead lines with Ona BTX-A was approved by the US FDA in 2017. The approved dosing for the forehead is 20 U Ona BTX-A, to be injected subcutaneously or intramuscularly at 4–6 sites across the forehead with intervals of 1.5–2.5 cm between the points. In men, the total dose of toxin could be raised to 32 U and at individual sites, 5–8 U of Ona BTX-A.

With limited sites of injection, toxin exerts its clinical effect partly through toxin spreading. However, adequate toxin spreading requires thinner reconstitution and is less precise in covering corners and recesses of the muscle. Fewer points of injection along with a high dose and more diluted toxin could achieve acceptable results in most patients, but this is actually a waste of toxin because of overfill near the point of injection and overlapping of two or more spreading territories, and it is not precise enough for fine adjustment and regional considerations. Diluted and large-unit toxin doses administered lower could result in overwhelmed suppression, interfering with eyebrow position and dynamicity (Figure 14.1a,b,c,d).

GLABELLA FROWN LINES

As the first FDA-approved aesthetic use of botulinum toxin A, treatment of glabella frown lines is the most common single-unit treatment. Traditional injection of the frown lines uses 5–7 points of injection, and 20–30 U of Ona BTX-A in total. Treatment doses can be as high as 80 U of Ona

DOI: 10.1201/9781003008132-14

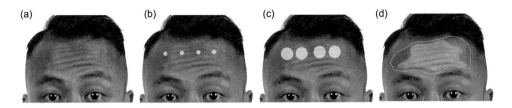

FIGURE 14.1   (a) Dynamic rhytids are variable in form and need to be treated individually. (b) Some procedures of forehead botulinum toxin injection treat the frontalis muscle with limited points of injection. (c) To cover the entire wrinkling area, the toxin has to diffuse adequately from the center point of injection; this can be achieved by large unit injection or diluted reconstitution. The clinical effect would be considered inferior if the toxin shows a diffusing tendency. (d) Individualized toxin treatment should be tailored to the muscle exercise pattern and magnitude.

BTX-A in men. Considering the small size of the targeted corrugator muscle, the individual point of injection receives a relatively high dose of toxin and one that is large in volume, according to the official suggested reconstitution. These two factors very much increase the risk of toxin spread to the neighboring muscles. Just as the limited points of traditional forehead injection after same reconstitution in similar units could suffice for forehead wrinkle control, a similar spreading of the toxin could happen in the glabella.

Full doses of the toxin administered to the glabella complex could freeze normal expressions and nonverbal communication. Unilateral deletion of the basic muscle tone toward the center would leave the remaining unopposed muscle pulling out and would widen the intereyebrow distance.

CROW'S FEET

Lateral canthal line toxin treatment was approved by the US FDA in 2013 with a recommended reconstitution of 2.5 mL. Two injection patterns were approved by the FDA, with a central injection point 1.5–2.0 cm lateral to the lateral canthus and bony orbital rim and two injection points 1.5–2.0 cm superior and inferior to the central points at a 30° angle. Each assigned point of the lateral canthus is injected with 4 U of Ona BTX-A. The lower injection points have to be kept superior to the upper border of the zygomatic arch and lateral to the vertical line passing through the lateral canthus. For those with lower distributed lateral canthal lines, the point above could be moved to the area between the central point and the lower point.

A 2.5 mL reconstitution and 4 U strategy all appear high in volume considering the very thin structure of the orbicularis oculi muscle. The widespread motor endplate (MEP) pattern of the orbicularis oculi actually allows the injector to give a more flexible and skillful touch to the lateral canthal region. Concern about impacting on the zygomaticus major can be lessened when the toxin is less reconstituted, the aliquot of toxin administered is smaller, and the injection is done more superficially (Figure 14.2a,b,c,d,e).

FREESTYLE INJECTION

The evolution of aesthetic toxin practice from the classical limited-point, high-dose injection to various kinds of newer approaches, involving more points and fewer units and being more flexible in terms of location, sometimes surpasses the practical requirements and verges on being randomly administered.

The originally restricted regime is often modified to lessen the unwanted full-block frozen effects. Most modern aesthetic toxin practices use fewer units to achieve similar effects. There are more and more theories about the application for popular indications deploying toxin in a freestyle way. Points and doses of injection are usually not well specified and could be easily adjusted according

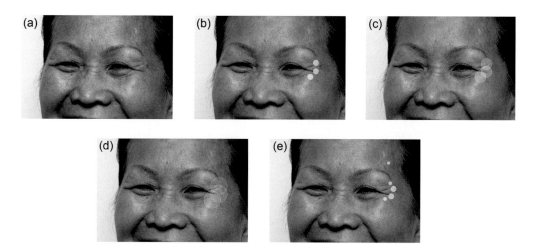

FIGURE 14.2 (a) The lateral canthal line is one of the usual aesthetic toxin indications. (b) For delicate control of the lateral orbicularis oculi activity, toxin working areas should be kept small according to individual conditions. (c) However, some protocols of toxin injection use doses and toxin concentrations similar to those used for the forehead. (d) What is effective for the forehead would have spread too much for this tiny area. (e) Customized treatment should titrate the dose according to the regional requirements and include touches to the neighboring structures to prevent any compensational distortion.

to personal will or in the name of so-called professionalism. Though local conditions of different patients based on clinical experience and visual evaluation require customized approaches, the toxin injections themselves should be plotted and counted in advance of the actual treatment, rather than being given randomly. The lower titrated dose in each point should be still quantifiable and documentable rather than trace amount according to wills impromptu. When it is hard to measure or record the exact sites of injection and the amount of toxin per injection, it is impossible to repeat the treatment on the other side to achieve areal symmetrical result. Sometimes the injection pattern is similar to the practice of microbotox but administered at bigger intervals, in doses that are a little larger, and injected somehow deeper.

Usually, the total dose given over the entire injection process is lower than the traditional protocol. The clinical result is claimed to be more natural. That could be imaginable because the average dose for a certain area of muscle is less. Muscles are not completely or deeply blocked. However, while these practices may look confident and skillful, some unavoidable problems remain behind the randomness:

1. *Standardizing problems*

    It is hard to record the injection points and doses, as everything that is done in a freestyle injection treatment is too random and doses fluctuate. When these patients return to be treated after the clinical effects disappear, it is hard to make the next treatment the same as the previous one. In other words, these kinds of treatment are not scientifically reproducible.

2. *Inadequacy and incompleteness*

    Because these random shots of toxin usually proceed quickly without visible postinjection tissue changes – except occasional and initial bleeding points – if there is no pretreatment planning, these injections easily overlap in terms of territory or cover the wrinkling area incompletely or unevenly. Superficial pricks and random shots leak toxins more through these punctures. Inadequate toxin dosing can result in short-term clinical effects, while incomplete treatment usually leaves residual muscle contractions.

These patients should be checked 1 or 2 weeks after the treatment, as second or more touch-ups are usually needed.

3. *Superficial effects*

These minimal doses of toxin are not easy to administer intramuscularly. The clinical effects of these superficial injections are usually through spreading from the superficial doses. The clinical results thus are usually claimed to be more natural.

4. *Asymmetry and imbalance*

It is usually alleged that freestyle injections can be tailored better to bilateral differences and regional muscular activity. Different doses of toxin are frequently given for corresponding bilateral points. However, most structures when compared to the opposite side are similar, with occasional obvious differences, although it is impossible for both sides to be completely identical. It is preferable that these subtle asymmetries in the bilateral structures of the face are not treated differently (see Chapter 8). Administering different doses through freestyle injections without a careful plan for adjusting bilateral minor differences is very risky as it aims to fill the subtle gaps but misses the gross bilateral equality. What makes things more complicated is that the random and complex unequalness is difficult to record and trace. Once again, a freestyle touch-up based on clinical examination 1 or 2 weeks after the treatment can correct the treatment. However, even if this second treatment is successful and achieves symmetry, it is not possible to reproduce this the next time.

5. *Immunological concerns*

Usually, freestyle toxin treatments need more touch-ups to correct minor asymmetry, inadequacy, incompleteness, and focal errors. Touch-ups and frequent toxin injections increase toxin immunogenicity.

INDIVIDUALIZED TREATMENTS WITH TOXIN

Aesthetic toxin treatments should be individualized, but they must be scientifically individualized. Every novel idea should be developed based on and evolving from the traditional protocols because of the documented evidence and experiences from numerous clinical studies and scientific data. Points of injection and dosing strategies should be tailored on an individual basis, weighing the subtle differences in anatomical features, muscle strength, possible asymmetries, habitual dynamics, and synergism that deviate from the standard protocol.

The recent advances in anatomy and neurobiology help us to modify further the injection pattern beyond the original dogma of restriction.

If the traditional teachings of points and units can be modified and improved in any way, it would be in the original purpose of treatment: to improve the status and morphological shapes, attaining a more desirable aesthetic presentation. However, the normally innervated muscle action, skin apparatus function or inhibition themselves have no direct relationship to aesthetics. The aesthetic enhancement from a treatment comes from intellectual design and selective moderation of the original muscle activities, changing the ways and shapes of presentation and making them pleasing to the eye, and recognition. Elegance and beauty are never the result of switching the apparatuses off or on. Any novel approaches must be able to be under control precisely between both sides and be reproducible to maintain the goodness.

BIBLIOGRAPHY

Ahn BK, et al. Consensus recommendations on the aesthetic usage of botulinum toxin type A in Asians. *Dermatol Surg* 2013;39(12):1843–1860.

Bertossi D, et al. Italian consensus report on the aesthetic use of onabotulinum toxin A. *J Cosmet Dermatol* 2018;17(5):719–730.

Carruthers J, et al. Consensus recommendations for combined aesthetic interventions in the face using botulinum toxin, fillers, and energy-based devices. *Dermatol Surg* 2016;42(5):586–597.

Lorenc ZP, et al. Consensus panel's assessment and recommendations on the use of 3 botulinum toxin type A products in facial aesthetics. *Aesthet Surg J* 2013;33(1 Suppl):35S–40S.

Sundaram H, et al. Global aesthetics consensus: Botulinum toxin type A – evidence-based review, emerging concepts, and consensus recommendations for aesthetic use, including updates on complications. *Plast Reconstr Surg* 2016;137(3):518e–529e.

15 Eyebrow Enhancement or Instability?

Yates Yen-Yu Chao

CONTENTS

Aesthetic toxin treatment began with the incidental finding that glabella frown lines decreased in the treatment for strabismus. The brow shape and position were also found to be altered in the treatment of upper facial wrinkles. Brow contouring is often listed as one of the many indications of toxin treatment for aesthetic purposes. In addition to the alteration of brow shape, botulinum toxin has been used for lifting, especially around the eyes. This chapter discusses the wisdom of using botulinum toxin for lifting and the pros and cons of toxin brow intervention.

BROW ANATOMY

The eyebrow is a hair-bearing area with a continuous compartment of fat (retro-orbicularis oculus fat) covering the superior orbital rim. In structure and in facial dynamics, this is an intricate area and a unit interdependent with the upper eyelid. There are several muscles working together in this area as synergistic partners or opposing components, pulling this piece of tissue in different directions through the skin connection. There are retaining ligaments in this location connecting the skin to the bone, but not exactly at the point of the hairy structure.

The frontalis muscle originating from the epicranial aponeurosis with insertion into the orbicularis oculi muscle complex (Figure 15.1) is innervated by the temporal branches of the facial nerve. A lifting vector is provided in accordance with the orientation of the myofibrils mildly aligning to the superolateral direction. The orbicularis oculi muscle has several origins, including the frontal process of the maxillary bone, the lacrimal crest, and the medial palpebral ligament inserting into the lateral palpebral ligament. The temporal and zygomatic branches of the facial nerve innervate the muscle. The most medial and lateral fibers of the muscle are arranged in a perpendicular orientation, pulling the eyebrow structure down with some tangential vector components directing to the lateral and to the medial (Figure 15.2). The depressor supercilii muscle can be viewed as a part of the orbicularis oculi muscle originating from the frontal process of the maxilla and inserting into the medial third of the eyebrow skin and the orbicularis oculi muscle. It helps pull the medial brow downwards and medially. The corrugator supercilii muscle provides most of the frowning force with its origin in the superciliary arch of the frontal bone and insertion at the medial brow to the skin and orbicularis oculi muscle complex. Innervated by the temporal branch of the facial nerve, it approximates the brow through the medial brow attachment in the inferior medial direction. The procerus muscle has its origin in the nasal bone and the transverse part of the nasalis muscle,

DOI: 10.1201/9781003008132-15

111

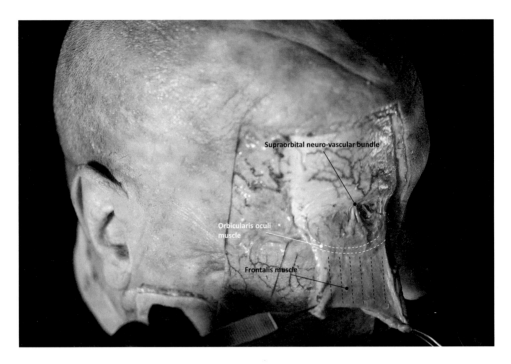

FIGURE 15.1   Cadaveric dissection of the glabella and forehead region after removal of the skin and sub-cutaneous fat. The frontalis and orbicularis oculi muscle are deflected to reveal the supraorbital neurovas-cular bundle, which emerges deep from the supraorbital foramen/notch. Neurotoxin migration through the supraorbital foramen/notch may cause eyelid ptosis by paralysis of the levator palpebrae muscle. (Courtesy of Sebastian Cotofana, MD, PhD.)

inserting to the skin of the glabella and the frontalis muscle there. It depresses the glabella skin downwards, with innervation by the zygomatic branch of the facial nerve.

TOXIN BROW LIFTING

The downward forces oppose the elevator action of frontalis muscle, mediating the position of the brow. Some studies found a 4 mm elevation of the eyebrow after weakening of the lateral orbicu-laris oculi muscle. While the medial depressors provide the force pulling it, not only inferiorly but also medially, blocking off the medial depressors breaks the harmony and reinforces the vector upwardly and laterally. That is why Spock's deformity occurs in several different scenarios when toxin has been injected in the frontalis or glabella complex. Incomplete treatments can result in unopposed pulling on the eyebrow superiorly and laterally (Figure 15.3a,b,c).

The brow position before botulinum toxin treatments reflects the relative strength of the brow elevator and depressors and the condition of tissue redundancy and laxity. Toxin treatment often creates an unopposed imbalance that elevates or pulls the brow. There are also some patients who have habitual imbalance among the opponent muscles that should be moderated with the toxin (Figure 15.4). The different muscles pivot at the structure of the brow, and lifting the brow lifts the eyelids as well. In patients with brow and eyelid ptosis, toxin chemolifting of the brow can improve the saggy appearance and open the eye apertures.

Where there is soft-tissue laxity and sagginess, the real problem underlying the tired and aging appearance is tissue redundancy and tissue looseness (Figure 15.5). Noninvasive energy-based treatments remodel the tissue and improve the quality with energy (Figure 15.6a,b); surgical trim-ming of tissue resolves the problem of redundancy without changes in tissue quality. However, in the

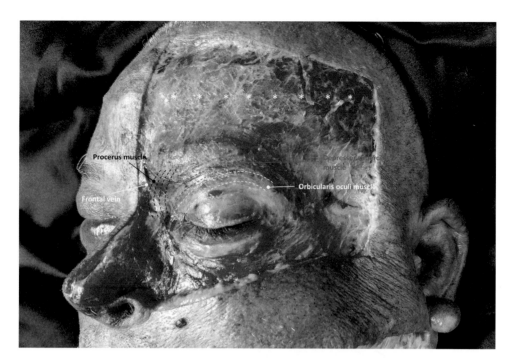

FIGURE 15.2 Cadaveric dissection of the left upper face. The muscles are highly interconnected with each other. The eyebrow and the frontalis muscle have no direct connection to the bone, allowing for high mobility. Please note how far lateral the frontalis muscle (*) extends. In some individuals, it extends lateral to the hairline. (Courtesy of Sebastian Cotofana, MD, PhD.)

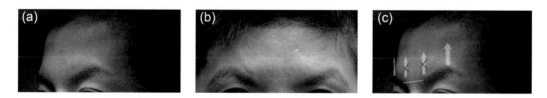

FIGURE 15.3 (a) Prominent elevation of the lateral hairy brow or an angular arch are less appreciated by Asian patients. (b) Suppression of the medial frontalis while preserving the lateral contraction distorts the eyebrow and upper eyelid dimension. (c) These mild forms of Spock's eyebrow are not desirable for Asian patients and resulted from unequal inhibition of the elevating net forces across the forehead.

case of toxin treatment, it is the fostering of muscle contraction – or, in other words, the imbalance between the brow opponent muscles – that moves the brow to a higher position and pulls the eyelid in consequence. The problems of tissue redundancy and tissue quality are not changed during this procedure. Conversely, the original normal balance between the brow opponents becomes unbalanced after the treatment. The subtle change in cases with mild redundancy and sagging might be considered an improvement. However, in cases with severe redundancy, tissue excess can hardly be sufficiently hidden through these muscle elevations. Redundancy and tissue laxity is a generalized problem not restricted to the eyebrow or eyelid. Forehead redundancy itself is usually exposed more in the form of folding wrinkles under a hypertonic frontalis. An irrational position of the eyebrow, an abnormally shortened forehead dimension, or distorted and sunken eyelids all complicate the path of correction that is not guided by pathognomonic considerations.

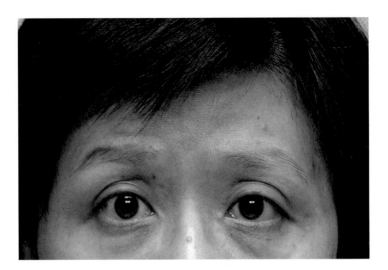

FIGURE 15.4   Habitual hypertonicity of the frontalis muscle is apparent in this woman, resulting in relative upper eyelid hollowness, inverted eyebrow pattern, forehead lines, and multiple traction dimples.

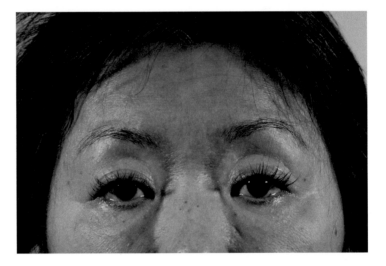

FIGURE 15.5   Compensatory elevated frontalis muscle tone occurs in many patients with eyelid soft tissue laxity and redundancy. The clinical appearance of these patients includes a displaced hairy eyebrow above the orbital rim, resting forehead lines, increased upper eyelid dimension and depression, sagging and droopy eyelid curves, and occasionally distorted eyebrow shape or orientation.

Neuromodulation should be considered in patients with hypertonic background contraction or imbalance of the eyebrow opponent muscles. The normal dynamicity of the upper face and a reasonable eyebrow position should be kept when applying toxin on the related upper face mimetic muscles for the purpose of lifting.

TOXIN EYEBROW RESHAPING

The shape of the eyebrow is the entire presentation of the distribution pattern, amount, density, and flow of the brow hair. Brow shapes often relate to local topography, the protrusion and shape of

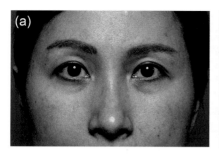
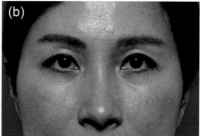

FIGURE 15.6 Frontalis hypertonicity is usually a subconscious response. The eye aperture, eyebrow position, and eyelid contour appeared more rested after energy-based treatments that raise the brows. (a) Before treatment; (b) after treatment.

bone, and the fullness of soft tissue below the skin. The eyebrow is a mobile structure pulled by surrounding muscles as a part of expression and communication. As toxin is used for the moderation of the muscles dragging this piece of hair up and down, the favoring of an upward vector is adopted as the treatment of brow lifting. Partial moderation favoring the contraction up or down is attempted to twist the brow into a different shape.

Spock's deformity might be criticized as an adverse result due to imbalanced dosing of toxin. It can also inspire novel ideas for crafting the turn and curve of a brow. However, if a raised brow is set as an objective of treatment by toxin intervention that breaks the balance among the opponents above and below the brow, a twisted brow that minimizes and complicates the imbalance would make the target even more unstable and less reproducible.

The orbicularis oculi retaining ligament helps maintain the position of eyebrows and to some extent limits their mobility as well. Pulling the brow up with an unopposed elevation drags it against gravity and away from its habitual attachment. The idea of turning a brow pulls the surface skin away from the alignment of the underlying ligament. The available muscles around the eyebrow, providing the vectors upward, downward, and a little medially, are not diversified enough to afford different shape selections.

The treatment of brow reshaping usually works with minimal doses of the toxin on a small portion of the muscle with the intention to minimally modify the interactions of the opponent muscles and minimally move the brow from the original position. Compared with toxin lifting, these minor adjustments are based on crafting toxin at specific points of muscle action with precise and minimal dosing. Local conditions of the brow vary among patients. The result of brow shape alteration by toxin is less predictable and more difficult to reproduce. A specific complex-patterned toxin-induced imbalance changes with time and is not easy to maintain. Minimal doses of toxin are aimed at a small portion of muscle and usually do not last long.

ADVERSE EVENTS RELATED TO BROW TOXIN TREATMENT

Limitations and concerns relating to toxin moderation of brow shape and position have been noted. Suboptimal results related to these practices are not uncommon. The most encountered problems relating to toxin brow alteration include the following:

- *Constant surprised eyes*
    The eyebrows and eyelids are raised above the neutral position to compensate for a sagging problem or an eyelid visual field obstruction due to unbalanced elevator function. That pattern of eye and brow shape mimics a surprised appearance but is presented in a more constant way. That contraction causes discomfort to the patient and interferes with facial communication.

- *Spock's deformity*

  This occurs often as an unbalanced partial brow elevation. Incomplete forehead treatment or unaccompanied frown treatment can both contribute to this effect. This strange appearance embarrasses the patient. It more often occurs in a relatively milder form, but it alerts other people that toxin has been used on the patient.

- *Aggravated forehead lines*

  Unopposed forehead muscle activity raises the brow and also folds the forehead skin more. Additional toxin to treat these lines should be given cautiously. The anticipated lift or shape soon collapses when the contributing muscle activity is stopped with minimal doses of toxin.

- *Paradoxical inner raising*

  Unbalanced brow elevation can happen in the opposite way to Spock's deformity. The appearance of this pattern of the brow is like a sad emoji. This often happens after an overcorrection of the lateral frontal activity and is accompanied by prominent central forehead lines.

- *Abnormal brow dynamicity*

  All the muscles targeted in treatments for brow position and shape are the mimetic muscles, which work coherently for expressions. The intervention of toxin in these muscles changes the resting state to one that deviates from normal. Expressions involving these muscles would certainly be affected in magnitude and pattern. This interferes with normal social facial interaction.

- *Brow asymmetry*

  Toxin muscle inhibition and compensation could be unequal and result in bilateral differences.

APPROPRIATE CONDITIONS FOR BROW TOXIN TREATMENTS

Treatments – whether for therapeutic or aesthetic purposes – should preferably normalize conditions that deviate from normal. Procedures that push these conditions further away from a normal or balanced state – even though they appear harmless or even effective – should be avoided as much as possible. Eyebrow alterations are valuable in several conditions like the following:

- *Hypertonic brow muscles*

  Hypertonic brow muscles are not rare. Patients who have had relentless frowning brows for years often have deeply indented static frown lines as well. There are patients with persistent raising brows as a habitual movement. Severe forehead lines are often the result of hypertonic frontal contraction. A compensatory hypertonic frontalis response can be observed in patients with eyelid sagging, and those trying to see through spectacles that keep sliding out of position. Hypertonicity can present as a partial activity in the central or lateral forehead or as a prevalent state.

- *Hyperactive brow muscles*

  This is the usual purpose of upper face toxin treatment. Toxin should be used only for moderation. In some patients, the focal hyperfunction should be treated with an additional dose aside from the standard treatments for upper facial lines.

- *Unbalanced or asymmetric brow muscle activities*

  Bilateral static hypertonic asymmetry or dynamic hyperactive asymmetry all need to be addressed with toxin to achieve a more symmetrical and balanced state (Figure 15.7a,b).

- *Pathological neuromuscular conditions*

  Injury or disease-related abnormal conditions could be considered for toxin treatment. However, practitioners and patients should be aware that toxin works by inhibition.

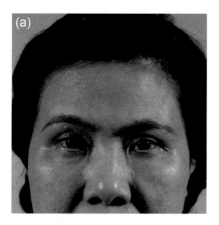 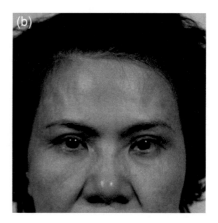

FIGURE 15.7 (a) This patient has been previously operated on for sagging upper eyelids, leaving over-wide creases bilaterally. (b) The asymmetric upper face presented with unequal forehead fine wrinkles; brow position, crease, and upper lid thickness were adjusted by toxin treatment around the eyes and on the forehead.

Abnormal neuromuscular activity can be adjusted through inhibition and made to look more symmetrical or natural in either a resting state or a functioning state, but it is not easy to achieve a good result for both states.

TIPS FOR BROW TOXIN TREATMENTS

- *Less dose for the first try*
  The toxin effect takes time. Toxin usually has exponential effects and these are less predictable on the first careful attempt especially for these focal adjustments. Practitioners should administer fewer doses initially.
- *Touch-up fine tuning*
  Before a solid regimen can be formed, patients who have received their first treatment need to be scheduled to return for a check-up. Satisfactory results usually need several touch-ups to improve the final effect. Additional doses and the points of injection should be well recorded.
- *Follow successful experience strictly through detailed recording*
  The second treatment should be much easier in the light of previous experiences. Treatment the second time should follow the first experience in order to put toxin in the right spots with the appropriate units. Successful reproduction of a treatment needs good documentation with photos and written records.
- *Adjust when conditions progress*
  When symptoms and severity change with age or after other treatments, the toxin treatment plan should be modified as well.
- *Be conservative and practical*
  Toxin treatment has its limitations. Severe and complex problems will need to be tackled with multiple modalities. Practitioners should refrain from endlessly pursuing effects with botulinum toxin alone.

BIBLIOGRAPHY

Chen AH, et al. Altering brow contour with botulinum toxin. *Facial Plast Surg Clin North Am* 2003;11(4):457–464.
Cohen S, et al. Forehead lift using botulinum toxin. *Aesthet Surg J* 2018;38(3):312–320.

El-Khoury JS, et al. The impact of botulinum toxin on brow height and morphology: A randomized controlled trial. *Plast Reconstr Surg* 2018;141(1):75–78.

Foster JA, et al. Modifying brow position with botulinum toxin. *Int Ophthalmol Clin* 2005;45(3):123–131.

Hexsel D, et al. Long-term cumulative effects of repeated botulinum toxin type A injections on brow position. *Dermatol Surg* 2020;46(9):1252–1254.

Redaelli A, et al. How to avoid brow ptosis after forehead treatment with botulinum toxin. *J Cosmet Laser Ther* 2003;5(3–4):220–222.

Schlager S, et al. A 3d morphometrical evaluation of brow position after standardized botulinum toxin A treatment of the forehead and glabella. *Aesthet Surg J* 2019;39(5):553–564.

Sedgh J, et al. The aesthetics of the upper face and brow: Male and female differences. *Facial Plast Surg* 2018;34(2):114–118.

Sneath J, et al. Injecting botulinum toxin at different depths is not effective for the correction of eyebrow asymmetry. *Dermatol Surg* 2015;41(Suppl 1):S82–S87.

Steinsapir KD, et al. Cosmetic microdroplet botulinum toxin A forehead lift: A new treatment paradigm. *Ophthalmic Plast Reconstr Surg* 2015;31(4):263–268.

Uygur S, et al. The quantitative effect of botulinum toxin A over brow height. *J Craniofac Surg* 2013;24(4):1285–1287.

Yoon NS, et al. Exploring brow position changes with age in Koreans. *Korean J Ophthalmol* 2019;33(1):91–94.

16 Refining Forehead Toxin Treatment

Yates Yen-Yu Chao

CONTENTS

Forehead toxin treatment is skill-intensive because of the forehead's unique anatomical structure and the confounding factors of the eyebrow and the eyelid that limit the consistent relaxation of this piece of muscle. This concern is greater in patients with aging-related sagging and redundancy, who are also the group of patients that need forehead toxin the most.

FOREHEAD ANATOMY

Horizontal forehead lines are the result of contraction of the frontalis muscle, which originates from the epicranial aponeurosis, inserting into the orbicularis oculi muscle complex. Movements of the frontalis muscle elevate the supraorbital skin and the eyebrow. Contrary to the traditional understanding of the forehead – as being below the frontalis muscle – there is a thin layer of deep central fat compartment bordered by the frontal periosteum, the posterior surface fascia of the frontalis muscle, the supraorbital neurovascular structure, and inferiorly by the middle frontal septum (Figure 16.1). Lateral to the neurovascular bundle is the deep lateral frontal fat compartment with a lateral margin made up of the temporal ligament. In addition to the middle frontal septum, there is a septal structure bordering the retro-orbicularis oculi fat compartment and situated below the middle septum as the inferior frontal septum. Superficial to the frontalis muscle are the superficial fat compartments that are bordered inferiorly by the frontalis insertion with the orbicularis oculi and procerus muscle and laterally and individually by the temporal ligament and supraorbital neurovascular structure. The superficial compartments can be divided into two lateral and one central, layered above the superficial frontalis fascia and immediately below the skin.

THE UNIQUENESS OF FOREHEAD TOXIN TREATMENT

The discussions on toxin spread, toxin concentration, and injection points are relevant for forehead toxin treatment because the intended muscle is broad in structure, the usual doses for the entire muscle relaxation are relatively low, and it is in proximity to the eyes, which should ideally not be

DOI: 10.1201/9781003008132-16

119

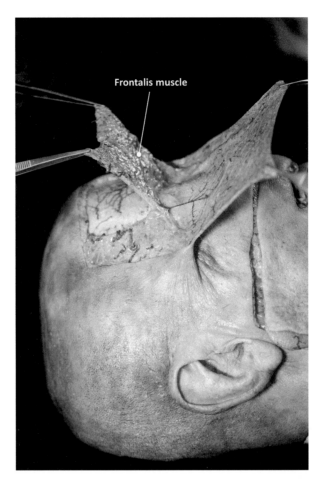

FIGURE 16.1   Cadaveric dissection of the forehead region. The frontalis muscle has no bony adhesion. It is located within a fascial envelope extending from the galea aponeurotica, the supra- and subfrontalis fascia. (Courtesy of Sebastian Cotofana, MD, PhD.)

affected. In a nutshell, the toxin applied here should be even and should cover the frontalis muscle as efficiently, completely, and precisely as possible.

VARIABLE FACTORS IN FOREHEAD TOXIN TREATMENT

Before starting forehead toxin treatment, injectors have to be aware of individual forehead conditions to ensure better judgment and design of the injection points and units of the toxin.

A. *Muscle pattern*

The frontalis muscle can have different structural patterns, with crisscross overlapping of myofibers in the lower middle, or not, and an empty window in the upper middle, or not. Some patients have tight brow tail skin interdigitation about the point of lateral thickening and can be noted to have a prominent depression when raising the brow. Arrangement of the muscle fibers results in a pulling vector vertically or laterally that can be assessed by visual observation and hand palpation when the muscle contracts. Though some forehead lines extend laterally out of the temporal crease, the frontalis muscle fibers are usually distributed within this landmark only. Toxin injection can be kept within this border, adapting to the muscle distribution and the presentation of forehead wrinkles (Figure 16.2a,b,c,d).

B. *Muscle strength*

The strength of muscle is related to the dose of toxin appropriate for muscle modulation. Muscle strength varies with gender and ethnic background. The individual differences can be assessed by hand palpation with the test of counteraction.

C. *Periorbital condition*

Normal brow mobility is part of facial expression. Some facial expressions involve the pulling of the frontalis muscle. Aging symptoms of the periorbital unit, including sagging and tissue redundancy, are more or less compensated for by the hypertonic tension of the frontalis. These intentional, subconscious, or background muscle activities will be blocked if the toxin is applied to the frontalis muscle. Heaviness or worsening of the upper eyelid and brow sagging are usually complained of by patients who have the problem of eyelid/eyebrow ptosis or eyelid tissue redundancy when toxin have been applied on the caudal forehead or in higher doses. Neutral eyebrow position, normal brow morphologic pattern, and dynamicity are often the result of a balance between the elevator and depressor muscles. Toxin treatment of the forehead could break this balance and result in some negative changes.

D. *Skin thickness*

Skin thickness, including the dermis and subcutaneous adipose tissue, varies a lot in the forehead area. Older people, females, and Caucasians usually have thinner overlying skin.

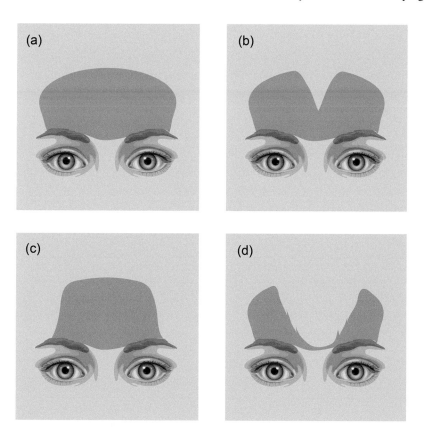

FIGURE 16.2 Based on anatomy findings, the shapes of the frontalis muscle have been classified as (a) full, covering the entire forehead; (b) V-shaped, with two separated bands and central aponeurotic tissue; (c) a central band with lateral aponeurotic tissue; and (d) a lateral form with a large area of central aponeurosis.

When forehead toxin is injected superficially, especially in patients with thicker skin, the superficially administered toxin has to spread across the skin to work on the underlying muscle. This would delay the toxin effect, decrease the clinical efficacy, and consume more toxin.

E. *Filler candidates*

As more and more injectable fillers are combined with toxin, the impact of fillers on toxin treatment should be emphasized in patients who have been treated with fillers or are going to be topped up with fillers.

If the fillers for the forehead are injected superficially to the frontalis muscle, the after-treatment thickness of the skin will be different. Toxin injected in a superficial way will have to travel longer to reach the muscle. Toxin wheals that result from superficial injection as toxin deposits in the dermis or subcutis as a pool will be instilled into the foreign filler instead. For the practice of intramuscular injection, practitioners have to adjust the depth of needle insertion according to the new thickness. The spreading pattern of toxins can change with the involvement of filler materials. A hydrophilic gel could redistribute the pinpoint shot well while a complex material and fibrotic tissue from biostimulation might perform like a barrier.

Multiple needle penetrations across the filler layer to muscle create multiple breaks in the skin. The mixing of fillers and toxins means that injectors have to be vigilant to keep all injections at a higher standard of sterilization.

The toxin can also have an impact on the effects of fillers, too. The toxin could release the frontalis muscle and decrease muscular activity, that interfers with the initial stage of an even filler distribution. Fillers that inflate the forehead contour or thicken the forehead soft tissue improve the appearance of forehead wrinkles and synergize the effect of the toxin.

STUDIES OF SWEATING TEST

The effect of toxin on the muscles has been studied through the simulation of sweating inhibition. However, the results and conclusions can be misleading.

Botulinum toxin is mostly used for myoneural inhibition and only minorly for sweating control of the same neural transmitter. When the toxin is injected into the forehead, our purpose is to inhibit muscle function, not sweat gland secretion. The frontalis muscle and the forehead eccrine glands are distributed at different layers. When forehead injection behavior is heterogenous, the scenario behind these attempts in the studies reported could be (Figure 16.3):

1. An intramuscular injection intending for a muscular effect
2. An intradermal injection intending for a muscular effect
3. An intradermal injection intending for a dermal effect
4. An intramuscular injection intending for a dermal effect

For a stratified structure with multiple layers of tissue, all the above conditions can occur. Some of the sweat gland studies reported did not specify the depth of injection. Even an injection with a trimmed needle cape to the control injection depth controls the depth of needle penetration in millimeters, this technique controls the depth in millimeter, not in a certain tissue layer. In another word, the same depth of penetration could reach different layers of tissue in patients with thick or thin skin. Whether the real penetration of the cuffed needle occurs within the dermis, the superficial subcutis, the muscle, the retro-frontalis fat, above or below the deep frontal fascia, is more related to individual skin thickness. The thickness of forehead skin indeed varies a lot in patients of different demographic backgrounds and usually is not controlled in most of these reported diffusion studies.

When the issue of the injection depth is controlled, can the extent of sweating inhibition by an intradermal injection explain the effect of muscle inhibition by intramuscular injection?

The tendency of toxin spread has been diversely observed in different studies (see Chapter 9).

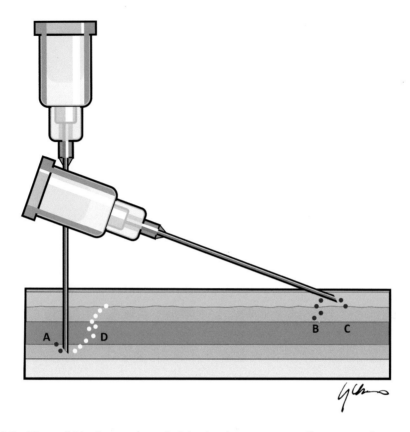

FIGURE 16.3 The antihidrotic exam by toxin injection does not necessarily represent the muscular effect. Sweat-gland inhibition requires that the available toxin be closer to the surface (C), while the injected toxin could be at a relatively deep layer initially (D). But the muscle structure we are interested in for inhibition is situated relatively deep. The toxin administered superficially (B) reaches the muscle differently from that delivered deeply (A). The difference might be minimal in patients with thin skin but will be prominent when there are longer routes of spreading.

WHY INJECTION DEPTH MATTERS

Even if we carefully examine the numerous reported toxin diffusion studies, it is obvious that the results and conclusions from the comparison studies across brands are not coherent. Injection depth is one of the key points magnifying the difference in toxin character. In a slim candidate, the entire soft tissue envelope overlying the frontal bone is extremely thin. In this case, whether the injection is deep or superficial does not matter as much as for the inhibition of sweating or muscle function. But in patients with thick skin, the injection at dermis would need to spread to the muscle to have effects but is more ready for subcutaneous sweat gland inhibition. In a similar way, a deep injection in a patient with thick skin has to spread back across the muscle to interfere with the sweating but approaches the muscle more easily. Attention to the toxin spread required by an injection will be more helpful in revealing the difference in diffusion tendency. For this purpose, we had the injections proceed in a pattern of superficial needle prick and vertical bone-deep depot to test the muscle effect and anhidrotic halo; we found that depth of injection matters (unpublished study) (Figure 16.4a,b,c,d).

The halo size obviously differs from superficial to deep injections. When our intended target is muscular inhibition, the accessibility of the target tissue will certainly vary with different injection depths. Since toxin treatment will be more efficient when the active molecule can be applied as closely to the target as possible, for forehead lines, the injection level should not be superficial, or if possible, be in the intramuscular layer.

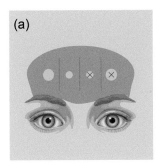

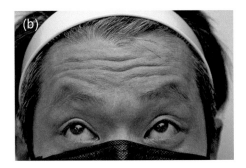

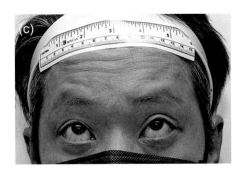

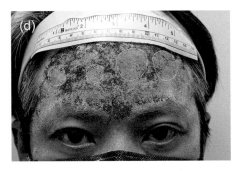

FIGURE 16.4 (a,b) Our study using concentrated low unit incobotulinum toxin injected through superficial prick (right of the patient) and supraperiosteal stab (left of the patient) is evaluated for anhidrotic halo and contraction inhibition (unpublished study). In this patient with normal skin thickness, surface toxin resulted in very limited muscle effect (c, left of the patient), compared to deep injection. (d, left of the patient) Deep injection of the same unit toxin resulted in a wider halo of anhidrosis.

TRADITIONAL INJECTION POINTS AND SPLIT DOSES

Though in these studies, the anhidrotic halo estimation for toxin spread in muscle is not completely compatible with the range of muscle effect, these haloesize – if arranged in the pattern of classical injection schemes for forehead lines – do not completely cover the entire forehead area. The halo size increases with increasing units per injection spot of the same concentration of toxin, increasing volume of the toxin with the same amount of active molecules, and increasing concentration of toxin when the volume of toxin is kept the same. But when the doses of toxin are elevated and the haloes become bigger, the toxin coverage is increased, but these big halos arranged in the same way still cannot flexibly adapt to the frontalis area. When toxin functioning diameter increases, the practice of toxin injection become less precise and more dangerous. This increases the chances of having unwanted impacts on the neighboring muscles. In other words, the method of increasing units per spot of injection or toxin dilution to cover a larger area is not preferred. Overfilling and wasting can occur in the center of large unit injection and also in the areas where two different large haloes overlap. For a better and tailored forehead toxin treatment, a split dosing plan, arranged according to the individual wrinkle pattern, condition of laxity, and structural geography, should be developed (Figure 16.5a,b,c).

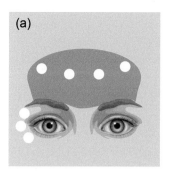 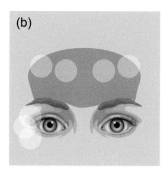 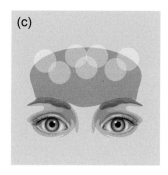

FIGURE 16.5 (a) The dose and concentration appropriate for small muscular units might cover broad muscles inadequately. (b) Dilution of the toxin can improve the clinical result by covering a larger area but could result in more unnecessary spread in smaller muscle units. (c) Increasing numbers of injection spots along with large unit injection or toxin dilution covers a broader area of muscle but results in more overlapping waste and awkwardness when it comes to fine adjustment.

CONCENTRATION AND TOXIN SPREAD

When a bolus of toxin fluid is introduced into the tissue, the initial existence of the fluid in tissue is actually adhesion hydrodissection. The hydrostatic pressure of fluid expansion through the plunger pushing forces the fluid to infiltrate through these intercellular spaces. The magnitude of pressure is related to many factors, including the speed of injection, total amount of fluid, tissue density, etc. The driving force of toxin spread includes hydrostatic and injection pressure – it is not purely the diffusion process described by Fick's law that molecules move from a region of higher concentration to one of low concentration.

For the same product, of the same volume, but with different concentration, the more concentrated one has a wider working diameter that is driven by the concentration gradient. For the same product, in the same concentration, but in different aliquot size, the bigger shot has a wider diameter of clinical effect. The increase both in volume and in active toxin molecules increases the functioning circle more than does only an increase in active molecules. For the same product, with the same amount of active ingredient, but prepared in different volume, the thicker one diffuses less (Figures 16.6 and 16.7).

The concentration of the injectable toxin fluid can be adjusted according to geometric requirements. Compared with the small muscle of the corrugator, forehead treatment needs more complete coverage. Forehead toxins should not be as concentrated as the preparation for delicate muscular structures. Forehead treatment plans can be modified in another way to include more points of injection when concentration of the toxin is kept the same.

TOXIN PRODUCTS AND SPREADING CHARACTER

Discussion on the relationship between the scope of diffusion and toxin concentration cannot be easily applied to everyday practice, as toxin products differ in terms of their manufacturing processes and their formulations. Though many studies on toxin diffusion tried to conclude that different products diffuse similarly when reconstituted with the same amount of saline, there are probably even more experiments that found them to diffuse differently. The many different studies set their conditions differently and the comparisons were not the target tissue but the structure ofsweat gland in a different layer; moreover, the tests were mostly on the forehead. Would it be too capricious to conclude that different formulations of toxins have the same diffusing tendency despite their considerable differences in manufacturing process, formulation, and reconsitution?

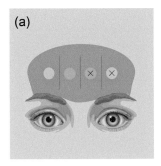
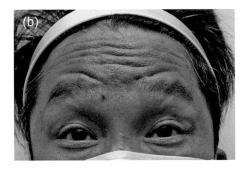
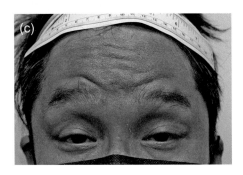
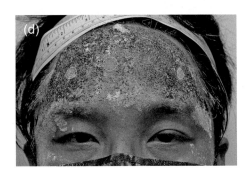

FIGURE 16.6   (a,b) The study on depth and concentration impact using incobotulinum toxin injected through superficial prick (right side) and supraperiosteal stab (left) is evaluated for anhidrotic halo and muscle contraction inhibition (unpublished study). In this patient with thick skin, diluted toxin was less effective (c, central) for muscle inhibition and functioning with a wider diameter when administered deeply (c, left of the patient). The diluted toxin with half the amount of toxin produces an anhidrotic halo of similar size when applied superficially (d, right of the patient) but cannot achieve visible inhibition when applied deeply in the lower unit (d, left of the patient).

The experiences of the author also point to the different diffusing behaviors among the different commercially available kits. Toxin diffusion tendency is an important issue for treatments of the forehead. If a toxin product tends to diffuse less – especially when forehead toxin is administered at 4–6 points of injection – it is highly possible that incomplete coverage due to lack of enough spread and a false lack of clinical efficacy will be perceived. When these patients are not closely monitored after treatment, they often come back earlier to request retreatment. However, a toxins of a greater diffusing potential, without careful preparation or dosing, can cause unwanted effects when approaching the eyebrows or eyelids. These uncertainties restrict its use for the lower forehead lines.

TREAT THE FOREHEAD WITH PRECISION

The toxin effect on the frontalis muscle cannot be as easily monitored from the anhidrosis test. Most clinical efficacy is evaluated by the calming of forehead lines. However, toxin effect assessment determined visually by the disappearance of dynamic lines is an indirect and imprecise measure. From the extrapolation of anhidrosis observation, it can be imaged that the frontalis is blocked in a pattern with residual activity between injection points. When these gaps are small, these residual contractions will be masked by the overlying skin. When these gaps become wider, there will be more visible residual contractions, and the results are usually regarded as incomplete.

When toxin injection is high in concentration or in large units per spot of injection, toxin accumulates and is wasted near the injection points, even though there is toxin spreading out within the effective circle.

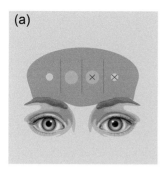
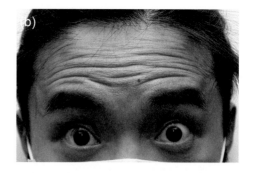
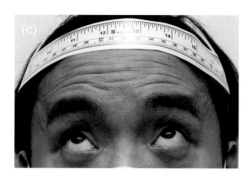
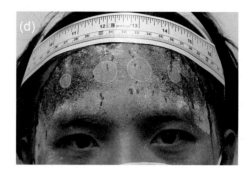

FIGURE 16.7   (a,b) Using small unit toxins with different depth and concentration of incobotulinum toxin in a patient with relatively thin skin revealed that the result of muscle inhibition is extremely small in diameter but larger and prominent in deep injection (c, left of the patient) (unpublished study). A small area of muscular immobilization is not easily measured as the folding of skin is continuous through the action of surrounding active muscle fibers. The measure of muscle effect by diameter measurement is extremely imprecise. (d) The diameter of the anhidrotic halo is similar in superficial and deep injection in patients with thin skin, but larger when the toxin is more diluted.

To refine toxin treatments that have to cover a wide muscular unit like the frontalis muscle, toxin injection can be administered with more points of injection but be smaller in aliquot size That helps to tailor the wrinkle distribution and structural pattern better. For the traditional forbidden area of caudal forehead, toxin actually could be administered as well but further refined as in a more elevated tissue layer, in more concentrated reconstitution, and with less toxin units.

BIBLIOGRAPHY

Anido J, et al. Tailored botulinum toxin type A injections in aesthetic medicine: Consensus panel recommendations for treating the forehead based on individual facial anatomy and muscle tone. *Clin Cosmet Investig Dermatol* 2017;10:413–421.

Arnaoutakis D, et al. Surgical and nonsurgical techniques in forehead rejuvenation. *Facial Plast Surg* 2018;34(5):466–473.

Cliff SH, et al. Different formulations of botulinum toxin type A have different migration characteristics: A double-blind, randomized study. *J Cosmet Dermat* 2008; 7:50–54.

de Almeida ART, et al. Pilot study comparing the diffusion of two formulations of botulinum toxin type A in patients with forehead hyperhidrosis. *Dermatol Surg* 2007;33 Spec No.(1 Spec):S37–S43.

Garritano FG, et al. Surgical anatomy of the upper face and forehead. *Facial Plast Surg* 2018;34(2):109–113.

Hexsel D, et al. A randomized pilot study comparing the action halos of two commercial preparations of botulinum toxin type A. *Dermatol Surg* 2008;34:52–59.

Hexsel D, et al. Field effect of two commercial preparations of botulinum toxin type A: A prospective, double-blind, randomized clinical trial. *J Am Acad Dermatol* 2012;67:226–232.

Hsu TSJ, et al. Effect of volume and concentration on the diffusion of botulinum exotoxin A. *Arch Dermatol.* 2004;140(11):1351–1354.

Jiang HY, et al. Diffusion of two botulinum toxins type A on the forehead: Double-blinded, randomized, controlled study. *Dermatol Surg* 2014;40(2):184–192.

Kerscher M, et al. Comparison of the spread of three botulinum toxin type A preparations. *Arch Dermatol Res* 2012;304:155–161.

Ozsoy Z, et al. A new technique applying botulinum toxin in narrow and wide foreheads. *Aesthetic Plast Surg* 2005;29(5):368–372.

Punga AR, et al. Biological activity of two botulinum toxin type A complexes (Dysport and Botox) in volunteers: A double-blind, randomized, dose-ranging study. *J Neurol* 2008;255(12):1932–1939.

Raveendran SS, et al. Classification and morphological variation of the frontalis muscle and implications on the clinical practice. *Aesthetic Plast Surg* 2021;45(1):164–170.

Ramirez-Castaneda J, et al. Diffusion, spread, and migration of botulinum toxin. *Mov Disord* 2013;28(13):1775–1783.

Renga M, et al. A personalized treatment approach of frontalis muscle with botulinum toxin A (Bont-A) related to functional anatomy: Case studies. *J Cosmet Laser Ther* 2020; 22(2):100–106.

Shaari CM, et al. Quantifying the spread of botulinum toxin through muscle fascia. Laryngoscope 1991;101(9):960–4.

Zhang X, et al. Botulinum toxin to treat horizontal forehead lines: A refined injection pattern accommodating the lower frontalis. *Aesthet Surg J* 2020;40(6):668–678.

17 Refining Toxin Treatment for Glabella Frown Lines

Yates Yen-Yu Chao

CONTENTS

Glabella frown lines were the first to be found and approved as an indication of the smoothing effect of botulinum toxin injection. They are also one of the most popular areas for botulinum toxin treatment for aesthetic purposes. With more and more understanding of their underlying structure and working mechanism, we can refine the management of frown lines better according to individual differences with better precision.

THE CRUCIAL ROLE OF THE GLABELLA

The glabella is a pivotal structure from both the morphological and functional perspectives. It connects the broad frontal space, the brow elevations, the sockets of orbits, and the nasal profile. Under the skin are complex interacting muscles that drag, twist, and squeeze this small piece of skin in different directions. It sits between the eyes and attracts most visual attention. The pattern of morphological connection determines individual features; this is the most important region for any portrait. Our eyes communicate and express nonverbal messages and emotions through the coordination of muscles around the eyes and brows that landmark the orbital area. Most of these movements involve the glabella complex. This explains the importance of proper moderation of the frowning unit for the purpose of reducing muscle activity that can be seen as communicating negative messages.

FROWNING TOXIN TREATMENTS

Most glabella toxin treatments target frowning. The frown is part of many expressions including anger, worry, discomfort, sadness, pain, and several others. It can be a response to external stimuli such as wind, light, smell, and others. Toxin treatment for blocking the glabella myogroup has been practiced since the start of toxin use in aesthetic procedures to reduce these so-called negative expressions. However, movements of the muscles here are not always negative. Some of them are neutral or even positive, like thinking, being moved emotionally, determination, etc. Treatments of the toxin that eradicate what are considered negative also leave this window of expression blank in other situations.

DOI: 10.1201/9781003008132-17

The normal response of frowning in patients as a part of their repertoire of facial expressions should not be blocked totally. In patients with habitual hyperactive frowning, responses can be moderated with toxin to reduce the magnitude of muscle activity. In patients with deep and stationary lines secondary to habitual muscle contractions, the toxin dose usually has to be high to achieve any significant correction.

DYNAMIC FOLDS AND PERMANENT LINES

Facial mimetic muscles, unlike other voluntary muscles that are attached to tendons or bones and contract resulting in the movement of the joints, are attached to the surface skin and can move the overlying skin, resulting in facial movements. These muscle contractions shorten the multilayered skin space, compressing them so that they fold as dynamic wrinkles. In areas where muscle contraction and skin compression are frequent, static lines gradually develop into permanent changes.

The origin and insertion of facial mimetic muscles can be connected to the bone, ligaments, or undersurface of the skin or interdigitate with another muscle. The depth of the muscle and the relation of the muscle to the entire layered structure have an impact on the capacity of a muscle to compress the overlying skin. Along with the thickness, turgor, and elasticity of the skin, contraction of the muscles results in wrinkles of different depth and intervals, but these are usually perpendicular to the contraction vector.

SYNERGISM OF MUSCLE IN FACIAL EXPRESSIONS

Although mimetic muscles are voluntary muscles, the recruitment of muscles to perform a certain facial movement is sometimes involuntary. A group of muscles simultaneously work together to complete a facial movement like a smile. Muscle activities are visible; surface electromyography (EMG) can be recorded with central peaks in crosscorrelograms. Common synaptic drives and functional synergy are proposed as the reason for the hard-wired repertoire of muscle synergisms.

Distinct voluntary and emotional pathways appear to exist for the facial nucleus innervation. Some voluntary responses are a learned process and some are hereditary pathways so that these nonverbal communications and responses are similar and understandable between individuals. Biological reflexes and reactions are to some extent inherent; our learning processes further equalize the pattern between subjects.

The glabella muscles work in cooperation with muscles outside the glabella to produce facial expressions such as a frown. This synergism is not separable by voluntary control. However, careful observation of these simultaneous contractions can reveal individual subtle variations.

When administering botulinum toxin treatments to synergic muscle groups, practitioners should bear in mind the cooperative phenomenon, and reasonable attention must be given to other members of the group to avoid compensatory hyperfunction of any overlooked muscle (Figures 17.1, 17.2).

ANTAGONISM OF THE GLABELLA MUSCLES

With different muscles pulling in different directions, some muscles act in opposition to each other, while some of the pulling vectors counteract each other partially. The eyebrow is a structure linked with several mimetic muscles as a pivotal area as well. Blocking one of these muscles actually breaks the counteracting balance and strengthens the muscle pulling in the opposite direction.

FROWNING PATTERNS

Frown-line toxin treatment has been generally administered in the standard way based on anatomical understanding and targeting the contributing muscles. Though dosages of toxin are titrated according to muscle activity, gender, and ethnic background, and injection depth can be variable

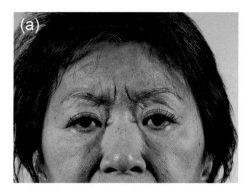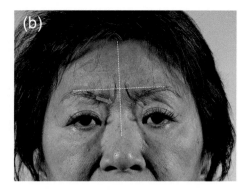

FIGURE 17.1   (a) The corrugator muscle contracts during frowning. (b) The orientation of corrugator pulls the hairy brow medially and a little downward.

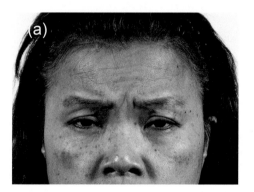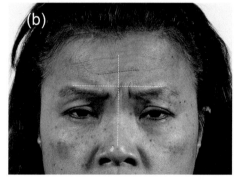

FIGURE 17.2   (a) Forehead lines appear in some patients when they frown. (b) The corrugator muscle and the frontalis muscle work synergistically in this pattern of frown.

based on age, gender, skin thickness, and physical properties, it is best practice in frown line toxin management to tailor treatment individually from a functional perspective rather than only taking structural considerations into account.

Different classification systems have been proposed based on the observation of dynamic wrinkle patterns. The different contraction patterns when people frown demonstrate the variant patterns of muscle synergism. The different classification systems share some similarities, but the ranking of prevalence shows distinct patterns when one compares the studies for Asians and Westerners (Figure 17.3).

A. *U pattern*

This is the usual pattern of muscle contraction when people frown. The whole process involves depression of the space and approximation of the brow. Muscles that approximate the brows and depress the glabella are involved. The frown pattern is identified by the parallel vertical lines between the brows and the horizontal lines at the nasal root.

B. *V pattern*

This is similar to the U pattern but has stronger muscle strength. All these combinations result in closer approximation, especially for the lower end of the glabella, the confluent zone of pulling vectors.

C. *"Converging arrow" pattern or 11 pattern*

Without horizontal creases or glabella depression, this pattern of frowning consists only of the approximation of brows. The procerus muscle can be quiet during the whole process

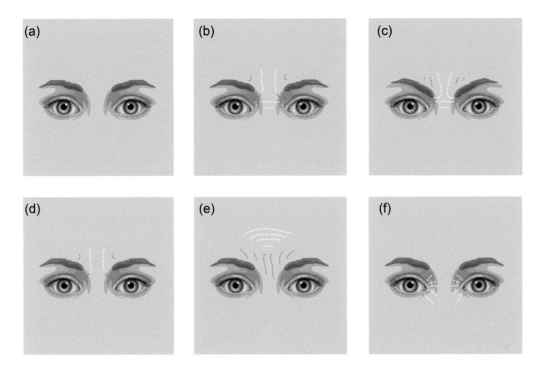

FIGURE 17.3 The glabella complex and neighboring muscles work together to produce the usual patterns of frown: (a) U type; (b) V type; (c) 11 type; (d) Pi type. (e) Medial orbital and perinasal lines often accompany frowning lines due to (f) the medial muscle fibers near the nasal root.

or in balance with the frontalis pulling force. In fact, there is also a balance between the frontalis and the corrugator's downward force to keep the glabella position stable.

D. *"Omega" pattern or "Pi" pattern*

When brows approximate in the frowning process, the medial frontalis fibers are also engaged. Their movements raise the medial brows and create horizontal frontal lines as well. The orbicularis oculi muscle is usually involved as well and not limited to the medial fibers.

E. *"Inverted omega" pattern or X pattern*

In addition to the engagement of glabella complex muscles, mid-face muscles also participate in the movement. The nasalis muscle is mentioned most for this combination. However, the lower part of the orbicularis oculi fibers and the levator muscles could play a role as well.

F. *W pattern*

This subtype based on morphological description of lines is actually a V frown with multiple foldings.

G. *I pattern*

In patients with thick skin, the 11 frown or the U pattern can present with a single line only.

Classification based on morphological observation is intended to reason and categorize the underlying muscle synergic pattern. However, not all muscle activities are revealed as the apparent arrangement of visible lines. The line patterns can even resemble each other when the actual contraction patterns are alike, for example, the absence of horizontal neck lines but presence of vertical muscle activity by palpation. The real activity under the skin and the relative magnitude of muscle strength should be carefully assessed individually to form a practical plan.

INJECTION STRATEGIES

Patterns of contraction suggest the underlying combination of muscle engagement. The injection plan should be based on the theoretical working groups of each pattern.

A. *U pattern*

Typically, corrugator and procerus muscles (Figures 17.4, 17.5) are considered the main players in a U frown, and injection could follow the traditional 5-point protocol.

B. *V pattern*

Orbicularis oculi is considered to participate in the whole process of a V frown, unlike with the U, but in fact the medial fibers of the orbicularis oculi are engaged in both patterns of contraction as eyelid movement can be seen in both. Additional superficial touches can be administered for the orbicularis oculi fibers. The stronger force of the muscle contraction in a V frown should be tackled with higher doses of toxin.

C. *11 pattern*

Toxin can be administered for the corrugator only in 2 or 4 points. Sometimes toxin has to be given superficially for the medial fibers of the orbicularis oculi when muscle activity is observed over the medial eyelid corner. The procerus point of injection in the standard

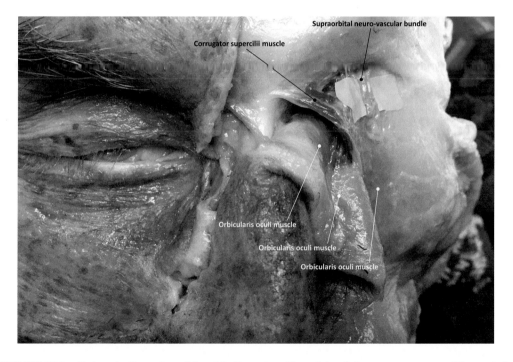

FIGURE 17.4 Cadaveric dissection of the glabella region. The origin of the corrugator supercilii muscle is medial to the supraorbital foramen at the supraciliar arch of the frontal bone. The supraorbital neurovascular bundle emerges deep from the supraorbital foramen/notch. Neurotoxin migration through the supraorbital foramen/notch may cause eyelid ptosis by paralysis of the levator palpebrae muscle. (Courtesy of Sebastian Cotofana, MD, PhD.)

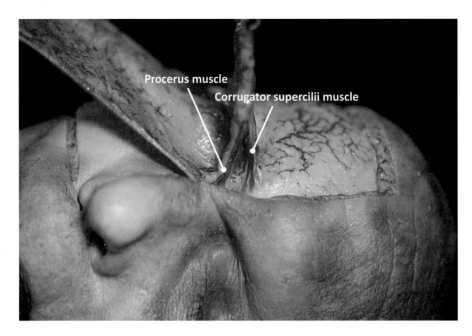

FIGURE 17.5 Cadaveric dissection of the glabella region. Note the bony origin of the procerus and corrugator supercilii muscle. (Courtesy of Sebastian Cotofana, MD, PhD.)

protocol is unnecessary and can make things worse when the tensional balance is kept between frontalis and the downward force. Injectors should keep in mind that the corrugator pulls the brows not only medially but also slightly downward. Injecting only on the corrugator inhibits brow approximation and raises the brow slightly, enhancing the upward opposing forces. A preventive minimal dosing can be considered to beadded if necessary.

D. *Omega pattern*

   In addition to the usual practice of injection on the glabella muscle complex, additional doses of toxin should be applied to the medial frontalis muscle. Minimal doses of toxin can be injected to the orbicularis oculi corners for a more elegant look. Frontal injection should be moderate, to keep the balance between the medial and lateral portions of the forehead.

E. *X pattern*

   Toxin should be applied not only to the glabella muscles but also minimally to the nasalis or mid-face muscles. It is suggested that the procerus injection be higher in dosage, and the balance between the brow depressors and the frontalis should be carefully preserved. The treatment regimen should be tailored according to the actual muscular contraction pattern rather than being determined by morphological line classification. The frowning classification system could be a formula on which to base further refined injection. Thorough consideration should be given to the opponent muscles outside the glabella to prevent unopposed neighbor hyperfunction (Figure 17.6).

GLABELLA TREATMENT PEARLS

Muscular synergism should always be kept in mind for aesthetic toxin treatment, and not only for the glabella. Imbalance between the opponent muscles should be avoided especially when muscular activities are to be suppressed but are originally in an active but balanced state.

   Although most injection protocols list the muscles that are involved in the whole process of a movement, the activity among the many participants varies. The actual regimen in terms of the number of units for individual muscles should still be left for the practitioner to calculate.

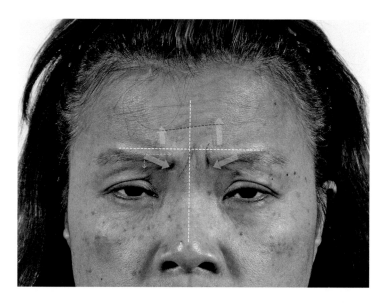

FIGURE 17.6 Corrugator muscle pulls the brows down and medially while the frontalis muscle pulls the brows up to counteract the downward pulling force. The left side frontalis fibers pull more and elevate the brow higher. The unequal activity of the frontalis drags the forehead and glabella skin into a deviated Pi, although there are no visible horizontal lines at the nasal root. Procerus activity may be present but is offset by the frontalis force. Palpation of the procerus area can detect subclinical muscle contraction.

The pattern of line distribution reflects only a part of the muscle activity. In patients with photoaging or deep engraved static lines, the morphological pattern can be misleading and interfere with dosing judgment.

The real purposes of glabella frown line treatment by botulinum toxin are:

- To decrease the amount, extent, and severity of frowning lines in order to decrease the intensity of expressing messages or emotions associated with a frown;
- To alter the pattern of frowning movement for more graceful facial dynamics and presentation;
- To balance the activities of this area with other parts of the face, especially when other facial zones have been treated.

The purpose of glabella toxin treatment is never to annihilate all the movements of this area or to erase the expressions or emotions from the face.

Keeping the variant patterns of frowning in mind, injectors should not fit their patients into some fixed program, giving doses as a routine, but should closely observe their patient's pattern of motions and strength of muscle movements by careful visual and palpable observation.

BIBLIOGRAPHY

Cho Y, et al. Ultrasonographic and three-dimensional analyses at the glabella and radix of the nose for botulinum neurotoxin injection procedures into the procerus muscle. *Toxins* 2019;11(10):560.

Cotofana S, et al. Respecting upper facial anatomy for treating the glabella with neuromodulators to avoid medial brow ptosis – A refined 3-point injection technique. *J Cosmet Dermatol* 2021;20(6):1625–1633.

de Almeida ART, et al. Glabellar contraction patterns: A tool to optimize botulinum toxin treatment. *Dermatol Surg* 2012;8(9):1506–1515.

Elghblawi E, et al. Exaggerated lower frontalis and glabella after Botox injection. *J Cosmet Dermatol* 2021;00:1–3.

Jiang H, et al. Different glabellar contraction patterns in Chinese and efficacy of botulinum toxin type A for treating glabellar lines: A pilot study. *Dermatol Surg* 2017;43(5):692–697.

Kamat A, et al. An observational study on glabellar wrinkle patterns in Indians. *Indian J Dermatol Venereol Leprol* 2019;85(2):182–189.

Kim HS, et al. A study on glabellar wrinkle patterns in Koreans. *J Eur Acad Dermatol Venereol* 2014;28(10):1332–1339.

Kim L, et al. Controversies in contemporary facial reanimation. *Facial Plast Surg Clin North Am* 2016;24(3):275–297.

Lee HJ, et al. Three-dimensional territory and depth of the corrugator supercilii: Application to botulinum neurotoxin injection. *Clin Anat* 2020;33(5):795–803.

Tipples J, et al. The eyebrow frown: A salient social signal. *Emotion* 2002;2(3):288–296.

18 Refining Toxin Treatment for the Masseters

Yates Yen-Yu Chao

CONTENTS

Botulinum toxin has been widely used for masseteric hypertrophy, which is usually idiopathic and can be attributed in some cases to bruxism and habitual jaw clenching. The prevalence of the masseteric hypertrophic problem appears greater in some areas like Korea. Genetic factors and dietary habits are postulated to be the reason. However, the configuration of Asian faces compared with those of Westerners – a wider dimension, a shorter longitudinal axis, a flatter front, and less anterior projection – could benefit from toxin block of the masseter muscles even if the size of the muscle is within the normal range. The reasons behind the wide facial and skull shape are partially genetic. Cultural baby-raising habits and sleep postures can have impacts on skull development as well. Along with the thicker skin and higher amount of subcutaneous fat, the facial shape of Asians presents predominantly in a rather wide and round format. The lower portion of a short square or round face often has problems of poor definition, a vague mandibular angle, and a continuous fat contour from cheek to neck. A round facial shape and cheek chubbiness, resembling the features of children, usually looks younger in adulthood and is considered more resistant to aging in appearance. However, the wide frame conflicts with the structure of the ideal facial profile; the childish pattern is not desirable after a certain age and hampers the features of sexual dimorphism. The mandibular structure is important in demonstrating traits of gender. Fat accumulation or masseteric hypertrophy all interfere with the presentation. Wide lower facial dimensions due to a bigger masseter distort the shape of the face further from the general preference for oval or heart shapes. The lower face is probably the only area of the face that can be easily modified in width and height when facial shape optimization is indicated. Masseter toxin moderation is an efficient and useful tool for holistic facial enhancement, especially for the lower face, and is not limited to people with real masseteric hypertrophy. Strategies for the lower face usually combine injectable fillers and toxin (Figures 18.1, 18.2a,b).

MASSETER ANATOMY

The masseter is the bulkiest muscle of the face, originating from the deep and inferior aspects of the zygomatic arch. The different heads of the muscle form the deep part and the superficial part (Figure 18.3): the deep part of the muscle inserts into the lateral aspect of the mandibular ramus, while the superficial part of the muscle inserts into the mandibular angle. A middle layer has been proposed for the insertion into the middle part of the mandibular ramus. The myofibers

DOI: 10.1201/9781003008132-18

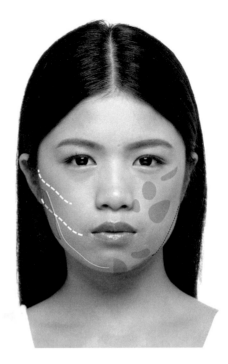

FIGURE 18.1 Filler and botulinum toxin are frequently and necessarily combined to tackle multifactor problems in a face, including those of the bony framework (white line) and soft tissue curves (whitish dash lines). A wide and square facial shape can be trimmed at the lower corners with masseter toxin (pink area) and lengthened at the tip of the chin, along with minor adjustments of facial contours (gray zones).

(a)

(b)

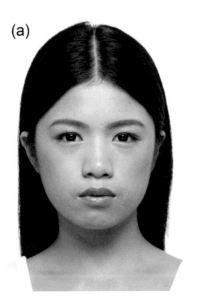
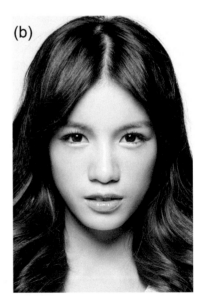

FIGURE 18.2 (a,b) Combination treatments with filler and toxin greatly improve the shape, projection, contours, balance, and interregional relationships.

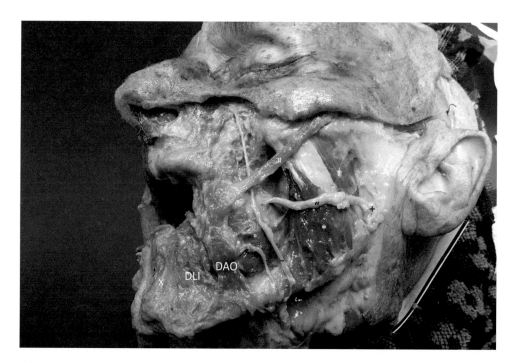

FIGURE 18.3 Cadaveric dissection of the mid- and lower face. The facial vein (blue arrows) and facial artery (red arrows) are exposed in the lower face, at the anterior border of the masseter muscle (*). The parotid gland (+) and parotid duct (") lay above the masseter muscle. The buccinator (°), zygomaticus major (#), depressor anguli oris (DAO), depressor labii inferioris (DLI), and mentalis (x) muscles are marked. (Courtesy of Sebastian Cotofana, MD, PhD.)

of the masseter are arranged in a pinnate pattern, which explains the strength of the muscle for jaw closure. Unlike the other motor units in facial and tongue muscles, which have fast-twitch fibers, masticatory muscles have substantial numbers of slow-twitch fibers. A heterogeneous distribution of motor unit types is found in masticatory muscles correlating with the heterogeneous activation patterns of these muscles. For the masseter, the proportion of slow-type motor units is larger in the deep and anterior regions for finer control and better resistance to fatigue, whereas the fast-type units are more common in the superficial and posterior regions.

MASSETER TOXIN TREATMENT IS DIFFERENT

Though masseter muscle toxin injection is still off-label, it is popular in some areas, even surpassing the official label uses. The target of the masseter muscle is functional for mastication, unlike the other facial uses on mimetic muscles that work for expressive movements. Sometimes the block for mimetic muscles is thorough and complete and the muscles after treatment are almost flaccid, but the masticatory muscle cannot be deadened completely. The masseter muscle has to be preserved for the basic functions of jaw-closing and chewing. As toxin is also indicated in patients with bruxism, trismus, masticatory muscle myalgia, and temporomandibular joint dysfunction, toxin for the masseter is not just for aesthetic purposes.

The masseter is much larger than most muscles that are treated for wrinkles, and the number of regular doses required for an effect on the masseter muscle is higher. In addition to the larger volume and the higher doses required, the masseter is thicker and compartmented in structure. The needle appropriate for this injection has to reach deep. The fixed needle on insulin syringes is too short to accomplish this in some patients. Deep injection of the masseter muscle has often been emphasized to avoid the spread to the risorius muscle, which has its origin quite superficially about the masseter and parotid fascia. Injection should be limited to the lower third of the muscle to lessen the incidental effect additionally on the risorius and parotid gland. The techniques of toxin placement in other mimetic muscles, which are superficial and delicate in amount, are not for the masseter.

TREATMENT EFFECTS AND PROGNOSIS OF MASSETER TOXIN INJECTION

The usual treatment of facial wrinkles with toxin has a clinical effect soon after the target muscles diminish their activity. However, the contouring effect of the toxin on the masseter takes longer. Most studies that measure the transverse facial dimension found maximum reduction after about 3 months. The long period of time that it takes for the measured size to decrease from the beginning of treatment explains the lower face slimming, as it derives not only from the gradual quieting down of the masseter muscle but also from muscular atrophy, which takes time.

Compared with the curve of various measurements about muscle size, biting force and electro-myographic studies show the greatest reduction at 2 and 4 weeks after the treatment, respectively. That shows that toxin inhibition takes 2 weeks to be complete.

The volume reduction according to various tools of measurement is about a 20%–30% decrease. Biting force decreases to a nadir at 2 weeks with a 20%–40% decrease and then gradually returns to normal about 12 weeks after treatment. However, complete volume restoration without further toxin takes 10–12 months.

Studies show that after repeated toxin blocks, the size of the masseter muscle can decrease a little further, but the decrease in biting force remains similar.

FREQUENTLY ENCOUNTERED QUESTIONS IN MASSETER TOXIN TREATMENT

- *Will these injections compromise the normal masticatory function?*
  The remaining function of the masseter and occlusal force are enough for most eating requirements. Most patients only feel the difference when they chew tough foods like beef jerky.
- *Will the other masticatory muscles have compensatory hypertrophy after the masseter toxin block?*
  Studies based on imaging observed no or minimal compensatory changes in the other masticatory muscles in human and animals after masseter treatment. However, there were reports of compensatory hypertrophy cases. Theoretically, this could happen when the remaining masseter function is beyond the daily requirement and when the muscle compromise has been prolonged. This means that our purpose in masseter block should be conservative, aiming to adjust the shape rather than to annihilate all muscle fibers. Practitioners should closely observe and listen to the patient about the function after treatment to keep the decrease in biting force within the threshold.
- *Why do patients complain about cheek hollowness after the masseter toxin block?*
  The tenting effect of our facial protruding frames lifts up the soft-tissue envelope, masking an underlying volume deficiency. A hypertrophic masseter bulges up the lower facial corners as ridges. However, soft-tissue volume can be deficient anterior to the hypertrophic muscle. When these patients are treated with masseter toxin without concomitant cheek volume restoration, the preexisting cheek volume deficiency will be revealed after the tent pole of protruding muscle collapses.

The hypertrophic masseter muscle provides support for patients with sagging jowls and a weak lower jaw. Filler augmentation should be considered at the same time to provide anterior structural support when toxin is to be administered to the masseter.

- *Why is toxin treatment not that effective in trimming the lower face in some patients?*

Toxin injected in the masseter has been well understood by the public as a treatment that can slim the face. However, a wide lower face could have different causes, such as a wide mandible bone. Patients with round faces often expect a slimming effect from toxin, but the roundness is usually the result of short bone dimension and a relative excess of fat. When the masseter muscle sits behind chubby fat or when the bone plays a dominant role, the volume change in a normal-sized masseter would not be very visible from the front (Figure 18.4a,b,c,d).

- *Why is paradoxical bulging observed in some patients after treatment?*

The masseter muscle is a highly compartmented structure. When toxin injection is limited to the deep layer, the superficial part of the masseter can remain unaffected even though the deep layer has been blocked. Fibrotic fasciae and compartment septa limit the spread of toxin. This paradoxical bulging is actually a compensatory hyperfunction of the remaining alert fibers. Toxin for the masseter should be administered through the thickness of muscle and to different compartments in the assigned region (Figure 18.5a,b,c).

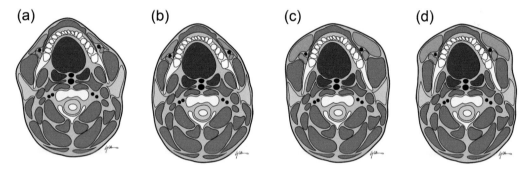

FIGURE 18.4 The clinical slimming effect of botulinum toxin on the masseter muscle is related to the underlying structural reason of the lower facial dimension. (a) When wideness can be attributed to muscle size, (b) the slimming effect can be prominent after treatment. (c) However, when the square dimension is the result of the bone shape or there is prominent fat-associated roundness, (d) the improvement can be limited.

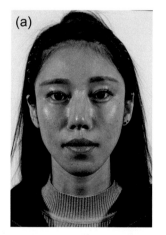
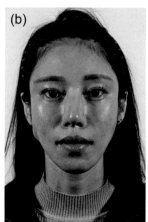
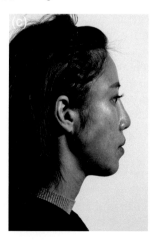

FIGURE 18.5 (a) After the masseter toxin treatment, there is prominent reduction of the lower facial dimension with residual minimal visible corner at the right side. (b) Paradoxical bulging is prominent at the lower part of the right masseter when the patient uses the masseter. (c) The remaining active masseter muscle belly is prominent from the lateral view.

PARTIAL TREATMENT OR FOCAL TREATMENT

The suggestion of preferential injection in the lower third of the masseter shows that toxin injection in different regions can have different clinical effects. Selective injection in the lower part of the masseter can preserve 70%–80% of the original biting force of the area without toxin administration. That is contrary to the classical neuromuscular theory about motor endplate distribution and muscle innervation. Actually, the endplates of muscle are distributed in a more versatile way than a middle bandlike structure. Some studies using multiple surface electrodes found that the endplate zone is not centered but spread out along the muscle fiber. This means that the usual toxin injection blocks only a part of the muscle, or, in other words, treats the masseter focally. Masseter toxin injection can further be selective for the posterior or the anterior portion, and involve the lower portion only or also the upper segment.

In addition to the recognition of endplate zone distribution, some anatomical studies find the arborization of the masseteric nerve looks denser in the middle inferior section under a special stain. However, the mechanism of toxin function is on the endplate neuronal synaptic membrane, not the nerve itself. Tracing the nerves is not completely the same as tracing endplates. When a contracting muscle fiber sitting further behind near the posterior masseter surface is to be calmed down, toxin molecules have to arrive at the endplates of that area. Though the nerve ending that reaches that fiber is branched from the hub near the middle-lower portion, injection of the toxin on the hub would not be effective for these fibers.

The usual treatment of toxin on the masseter, or the lower masseter, is usually not to saturation and, from the perspective of treatment purposes, it does not need to be total. This kind of partial treatment can become a problem when the untouched fibers are grouped together. Paradoxical bulging is one of these examples, having fascia or septa as a barrier to interfere with toxin distribution. Sometimes these episodes can be attributed to poor techniques indistributing toxin doses and limited points of injection to cover a big muscle.

ARTISTIC STRATEGIES FOR BETTER FACIAL CONTOURS

The masseter muscle is an important constituent of facial contour. It also has a role in cheek fullness; cheek transition curves; lower facial width; the geography, bulkiness, and angular pattern of the outward mandibular shape; and the frontal-view facial shape. The ultimate goal of masseter treatment is the shape, not the quietness, of the muscle. An artistic approach should be adopted when giving toxin.

Focal treatment is possible to tailor the injection better to fit the desired shape. But preferential dosing and selectivity should be optimized by a gradient difference between areas to achieve better smoothness. For example, for a patient who is slim or for those who dislike angles, it is not necessary to treat the entire lower masseter. Skin quality, the original soft-tissue volume of the cheek, the silhouette in front view and configuration of underlying mandible bone, the distribution and amount of nearby fat pads, gender, and the preference of patients should be all considered when devising a reasonable toxin treatment plan.

BIBLIOGRAPHY

Ågren M, et al. The effect of botulinum toxin injections on bruxism: A systematic review. *J Oral Rehabil* 2020;47(3):395–402.

Babuccu B, et al. The effect of the Botulinum toxin-A on craniofacial development: An experimental study. *Ann Plast Surg* 2009;63(4):449–456.

Hong JY, et al. Efficacy and safety of a novel botulinum toxin a for masseter reduction: A randomized, double-blind, placebo-controlled, optimal dose-finding study. *Dermatol Surg* 2021;47(1):e5–e9.

Kim DH, et al. Intramuscular nerve distribution of the masseter muscle as a basis for botulinum toxin injection. *J Craniofac Surg* 2010;21:588–591.

Kim HJ, et al. Effects of botulinum toxin type A on bilateral masseteric hypertrophy evaluated with computed tomographic measurement. *Dermatol Surg* 2003;29(5):484–489.

Kim JH, et al. Effects of two different units of botulinum toxin type A evaluated by computed tomography and electromyographic measurements of human masseter muscle. *Plast Reconstr Surg* 2007;119(2):711–717.

Kim KS, et al. Muscle weakness after repeated injection of botulinum toxin type A evaluated according to bite force measurement of human masseter muscle. *Dermatol Surg* 2009;35(12):1902–1906.

Lee HJ, et al. The anatomical basis of paradoxical masseteric bulging after botulinum neurotoxin type A injection. Toxins 2017;9:9010014.

Park HU, et al. Changes in masticatory function after injection of botulinum toxin type A to masticatory muscles. *J Oral Rehabil* 2013;40(12):916–922.

Pihut M, et al. Measurement of occlusal forces in the therapy of functional disorders with the use of botulinum toxin type A. *J Physiol Pharmacol* 2009;60(Suppl 8):113–116.

Pihut M, et al. The efficiency of botulinum toxin type A for the treatment of masseter muscle pain in patients with temporomandibular joint dysfunction and tension-type headache. *J Headache Pain* 2016;17:29.

To EW, et al. A prospective study of the effect of botulinum toxin A on masseteric muscle hypertrophy with ultrasonographic and electromyographic measurement. *Br J Plast Surg* 2001;54(3):197–200.

Xie Y, et al. Classification of masseter hypertrophy for tailored botulinum toxin type A treatment. *Plast Reconstr Surg* 2014;134(2):209e–218e.

Index

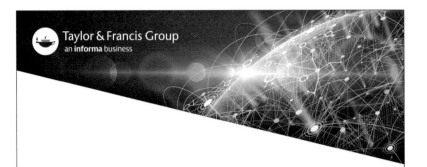